O9-BTN-126

NORTHAMPTON COMMUNITY
DISCARDED
COLLEGE LIBRARY

NORTHAMPTON COUNTY AREA
Learning Resources Center
Bethlehem, Pa. 18017
COMMUNITY COLLEGE

dying and death

an annotated bibliography

Irene L. Sell, R.N., Ed.D.
*Associate Professor of Nursing,
Long Island University*

The Tiresias Press
New York

With love and appreciation to
Selma Schumacher Smith

The Tiresias Press, Inc.
116 Pinehurst Ave., New York City 10033

Library of Congress
Catalog Card Number: 76-58052
International Standard
Book Number: 0-913292-36-2

Printed in U.S.A.

preface

The articles, books, and audiovisual materials annotated in this bibliography were selected for their relevance to and implications for nursing. While members of other caring professions interested in the areas of dying and death will find the bibliography useful, it was prepared primarily for nursing practitioners, educators, and students involved with providing care for dying patients.

The 506 annotations in this book are grouped into three sections: 382 articles in Section A, 71 books in Section B, and 53 audiovisuals in Section C. Materials within each section are numbered and cited alphabetically by author or title. The author and subject indexes use section letters and entry numbers to direct the reader to the citations.

The items annotated represent the work of nursing practitioners and students, nursing educators and researchers, social scientists, social workers, thanatology experts, psychologists, clergymen, physicians, creative writers, families of patients, the dying patients themselves, and others. Many of these materials were published in the 1960s, more in the 1970s, but materials judged relevant and/or frequently referred to in the literature are included regardless of the date of orginal publication.

The items included are concerned with the emotional, psychosocial, or interpersonal aspects of the dying situation and focus on the dying individual, his family, and/or his caregivers. Attitudes toward dying and death, communication patterns and problems, dying situations, sudden infant death, pain relief, grief, stages of dying, and nursing care of the dying are a few of the many topics covered. An effort was made to select materials that will contribute to the nurse's theoretic knowledge and/or that have a potential for practical application in the clinical situation.

Through cross-referencing and succinct annotation, this book reduces searching time. If a needed journal is not readily available, the entry indicates whether the article can be found in another journal or in a collection of reprints. In addition, pertinent contributions from books of collected papers that are cited in Section B are annotated in Section A, another short-cut for the reader.

It is the author's hope that this bibliography will help to guide all who work with dying patients to information they can use to enhance their knowledge and understanding of dying and death, and to better care for the dying patients and their families that they have made a commitment to serve.

I.L.S.

section A
articles

Section A consists of annotations of articles that have appeared in journals or in publications of collected papers. Standard bibliographic format is used in the citations. However, when the source of an article in Section A is annotated in Section B (the book section), an abridged citation is used to prevent the repetition of data. For example, Entry A-18, "If You Were Dying. . .," was originally published in a book that is annotated in Section B. This fact is noted as follows:

18. ASSELL, Ruth A. " If You Were Dying. . .," in *The Dying Patient: A Supportive Approach,* pp. 47-71 (B-8).

The reader who wishes to know the name of the book's editor or publisher or the date of publication can find that information in Entry B-8.

When an article cited in Section A can be found in an additional source, the words "Also in" precede the name of that source. If the second source is annotated in Section B, the reader is referred to the Section B entry number.

The bibliographic data on articles that can be obtained from organizations are concluded with the words "Available from," followed by the name of the organization. Requests for such material usually are made through local chapters, but the national office of the organization can be contacted for information if necessary. The addresses of the national offices of organizations mentioned in Section A are:

American Cancer Society, 777 Third Avenue, New York City, NY 10017

Euthanasia Educational Council, Room 831, 250 West 57th Street, New York City, NY 10019

The National SIDS Foundation, Room 1904, 310 South Michigan Avenue, Chicago, IL 60604

1. ABRAMS, Ruth D. "The Patient with Cancer – His Changing Pattern of Communication." *New England Journal of Medicine,* 274:317-322, February 10, 1966.
Social worker's observations. Says cancer most feared disease. Discusses behavior and communication differences in initial, advancing, and terminal stages. Presents three clinical examples.

2. ______ . "The Patient with Cancer – His Changing Pattern of Communication." *Annals of the New York Academy of Sciences,* 164:881-896, December, 1969.
Content same as Entry A-1 except for omission of clinical examples and addition of audience/author comments following presented paper.

3. ______ . "Denial and Depression in the Terminal Cancer Patient: A Clue for Management." *Psychiatric Quarterly*, 45, no. 3:394-404, 1971.
Views denial and depression as major defenses patients use in communication patterns that change as disease progresses; exerpts from verbalizations and descriptions of behavior demonstrate these defenses in patient selected as "prototypical of the majority of cases studied." See Entry A-359 for critique.

4. ______ . "The Responsibility of Social Work in Terminal Cancer," in *Psychosocial Aspects of Terminal Care,* pp. 173-182 (B-52).
Comments on social workers' area of concern and ways they contribute to care of cancer patients and their families. Notes differences between cancer patients and those with other fatal diseases; how cancer patients use denial and depression as means of coping.

5. AGUILERA, Donna C. "Crisis: Death and Dying," in *ANA Clinical Sessions: American Nurses' Association, 1968 Dallas.* New York: Appleton-Century-Crofts, 1968. Pp. 269-278.
Comments on nurses' attitudes toward dying, death; patients' needs and reactions to dying situations; awareness contexts; nurses' need to recognize and discipline own feelings and attitudes to care for dying patients; nurses' composure tactics; family reactions to patient's death. Outlines mourning process; suggests viewing death and mourning in crisis intervention model to facilitate nursing action.

6. ______ . "Crisis: Moment of Truth." *Journal of Psychiatric Nursing and Mental Health Services*, 9:23-25, May/June, 1971. Condensation of "Crisis: Death and Dying," cited in Entry A-5.

7. ALDRICH, C. Knight. "The Dying Patient's Grief." *Journal of the American Medical Association,* 184:329-331, May 4, 1963.

Comments on arguments for and against telling patient he is dying. Uses circular diagrams to illustrate patient's anticipated losses. Discusses anticipatory grief and how grief is influenced by the quality of interpersonal relationships, use of denial, and extent of regression.

8. ______ . "Some Dynamics of Anticipatory Grief," in *Anticipatory Grief,* pp. 3-9 (B-53).

Contrasts anticipatory grief with conventional grief and discusses differences in relation to endpoints, acceleration, ambivalence, and denial.

9. ALVAREZ, Walter C. "Care of the Dying." *Journal of the American Medical Association,* 150:86-91, September 13, 1952.

Physician notes moral and legal responsibilities involved in determining how much to tell dying patients; discusses physician attitudes toward dying. Elaborates on supportive and helpful care approaches, intervention with families.

10. ANDREWS, Linda. "The Last Night." *American Journal of Nursing,* 74:1305-1306, July, 1974. Also in *Dying and Grief: Nursing Interventions,* pp. 81-83 (B-45).

Critical care nurse tells of personal decision not to start resuscitation measures on 72-year-old man.

11. ANGER, Diane and Daniel W. Anger. "Dialysis Ambivalence: A Matter of Life and Death." *American Journal of Nursing,* 76:276-277, February, 1976.

Identifies four areas of professional conflict which arise when a patient decides to discontinue life-prolonging dialysis. Notes staff members' need to explore their own feelings and values before they can support such a decision.

12. ANNAS, George J. "Rights of the Terminally Ill Patient." *Journal of Nursing Administration,* 4:40-44, March/April, 1974.

Lawyer indicates need for nurses and physicians to see that patients' rights are respected, preserved. Discusses a patient's right to: know truth; confidentiality and privacy; consent to treatment; choose place and time of death; determine disposition of his body. Cites 33 references.

13. ARMIGER, Sister Bernadette. "Reprise and Dialogue." *Nursing Outlook,* 16:26-28, October, 1968. Also in *The Dying Patient: A Nursing Perspective,* pp. 25-30 (B-6).

Comments on whether nurses should hasten a patient's death as implied by Shepherd in companion article, cited in Entry A-324. Believes Shepherd's arguments violate logic. Discusses hazards involved in deciding who is to assume responsibility for ending life when it is miserable.

14. ARMSTRONG, Margaret E. "Dying and Death – and Life Experiences of Loss and Gain: A Proposed Theory." *Nursing Forum,* 14, no. 1:95-104, 1975.

Outlines grieving process. From students' reports of nondeath loss experiences concludes associated behavioral process is similar in all types of loss. Offers guides for strengthening students' behavioral patterns for coping successfully with loss, including death.

15. ARONSON, Gerald J. "Treatment of the Dying Patient," in *The Meaning of Death,* pp. 251-258 (B-19).

Offers guidelines for communicating with a patient and helping him maintain hope, retain his identity and individuality. Says physician must give of self. Provides clinical examples of effective and noneffective physician intervention.

16. ARTEBERRY, Joan K. "Distance and the Dying Patient," in *Current Concepts in Clinical Nursing,* edited by Betty S. Bergersen and others. St. Louis: The C. V. Mosby Company, 1968. Pp. 128-136.

Comments on uncertain definition of death by examining who are considered dying patients; indicates there are no stereotypes, few universals. Notes factors influencing nurses' responses to dying patients, and explores use of distance as an interpersonal tool in therapeutic use of self.

17. ASSELL, Ruth A. "Existential Approach to Death." *Nursing Forum,* 8, no. 2:200-211, 1969.

Outlines ideas held by atheistic and Christian philosophers regarding death; discusses implications of divergent orientations for nurses caring for patients facing death.

18. ______ . "If You Were Dying. . . " in *The Dying Patient: A Supportive Approach,* pp. 47-71 (B-8).

Asks reader to imagine his or her own death to facilitate discussion about nurses' involvement with dying patients. Considers implications of awareness contexts for interacting with dying patients and helping them gain inner peace. Identifies nursing actions contributory to outer peace; offers suggestions for supporting patient's family; comments on home care situations and care of comatose patients.

19. AYD, Frank J. "The Hopeless Case." *Journal of the American Medical Association,* 181:1099-1102, September 29, 1962.

Discusses factors involved in deciding to institute or withhold heroic measures; distinguishes between ordinary and extraordinary treatment; comments on right of patients to accept or reject treatment, refuse life-prolongation, request life-shortening.

20. BADER, Madelaine A. "Nursing Care and Interpersonal Relationships," in *The Terminal Patient: Oral Care,* pp. 195-207 (B-39).

Comments on the professional nurse's need for disciplined intellectual approach combined with therapeutic use of self for effective nursing intervention in dying situations. Indicates how relationships among staff members influence patients' care and describes how the Crisis Awareness and Management Project (CAM) at Walter Reed Army Medical Center assists hospital staff in dealing with dying and death.

21. ______ . "Personalizing the Management of Pain for the Terminally Ill Patient," in *Psychopharmacologic Agents for the Terminally Ill and Bereaved,* pp. 202-211 (B-26).

Describes nursing care situation in which a dying woman with unrelenting pain participated in a care regimen in which she selected her own medication (from a list), evaluated its effect, and arrived at a combination that controlled pain and kept her alert.

22. BAER, Ruth F. "The Sick Child Knows," in *Should the Patient Know the Truth?* pp. 100-106 (B-58).

Believes it is not necessary for child patient to be told serious prognosis, but identifies his need for help in learning about his disease and managing truth for himself. Indicates influences on nurse's decision to tell or deny truth, noting why evasion is often used.

23. BAKER, Joan M. and Karen C. Sorensen. "A Patient's Concern with Death." *American Journal of Nursing,* 63:90-92, July, 1963. Also in *The Dying Patient: A Nursing Perspective,* pp. 82-88 (B-6).

Notes how nurses' experience and philosophy influence their responses to patients who express concern about death. Illustrates why many nurses, uncomfortable with subject, discourage death talk. Identifies three principles for discussing death and other emotionally charged subjects.

24. BARCKLEY, Virginia. "What Can I Say to the Cancer Patient?" *Nursing Outlook,* 6:316-319, June, 1958. Available from American Cancer Society.

Identifies cancer patients' fears that stem from situation realities, nurse responses and actions. Discusses what talking about dying and death requires of nurses, how expertise in communication makes honesty possible whether patients are aware or unaware of diagnosis.

25. ______ . "Enough Time for Good Nursing." *Nursing Outlook,* 12:44-48, April, 1964. Also in *Nursing and the Cancer Patient,* pp. 1-10 (B-7).

Describes Calvary Hospital, where comfort care is nursing goal and death is not considered defeat. Comments on training program for nursing technicians; nursing measures that promote comfort and dignity; nurses' involvement with families; importance of adequate medication.

26. ______ . "The Crises in Cancer." *American Journal of Nursing,* 67:278-280, February, 1967. Also in *Nursing and the Cancer Patient,* pp. 49-53 (B-7). Available from American Cancer Society.

Comments on how people view cancer. Discusses crises involving diagnosis and surgery for patients, crises families experience, how nurses can provide support.

27. ______ . "Grief, a Part of Living." *Ohio's Health*, 20:34-38, April/May, 1968. Available from American Cancer Society.
Notes tendency to equate cancer with death. Focuses on irreversible stage, on grief accompanying it. Describes many grief behaviors. Explains care concepts with analogy to the shielding, time, and distance precautions used in Xray.

28. BARD, Bernard and Joseph Fletcher. "The Right to Die." *Atlantic Monthly*, 221:59-64, April, 1968.
Grieving father of son born with Down's syndrome tells about emotional impact of decision to institutionalize neonate; pleads for direct euthanasia after visiting institution caring for severely afflicted victims. Theologian Fletcher supports view with critique of indirect euthanasia.

29. BARROCAS, Albert. "The Dying Patient – a Team Affair." *Surgical Team*, 2:38-43, July/August, 1973. Also in *Nursing Digest*, 2:62-66, May, 1974.
Surgeon views honest communication among health team personnel, family, patient as essential to provide peaceful, dignified death. Considers difficulties involved in determining whether to use or withhold lifesaving heroic measures.

30. BEAUCHAMP, Joyce M. "Euthanasia and the Nurse Practitioner." *Nursing Forum*, 14, no. 1:56-73, 1975. Also in *Nursing Digest*, 4:83-85, Winter, 1976.
Gives sketchy definitions of terms to indicate differences between voluntary and involuntary euthanasia. Notes ethical, legal considerations; outlines arguments for and against voluntary form; vague about implications for nurses. *Forum* article cites 19 references.

31. BECK, Rudy. "Helping to Make His Last Dream a Reality." *Journal of Gerontological Nursing*, 1:10-12, May/June, 1975.
Tells how rehabilitation nurse's success with bowel and bladder training program made possible a 62-year-old dying man's dream of trip to California before his death. Describes positive influence of this success on staff's care of other residents in nursing home.

32. BECKER, Arthur H. and Avery D. Weisman. "The Patient with a Fatal Illness – To Tell or Not to Tell?" *Journal of the*

American Medical Association, 201:646-648, August 21, 1967.

Clergyman Becker responds to request for guidelines in care of 62-year-old man unaware he has metastatic cancer with comments on honesty, areas for physician to consider, and clergy's concern with patient's relationship to God. Psychiatrist Weisman says central question is not whether to tell or not tell, but who, how much, what, how, when, and how often to tell.

33. BENOLIEL, Jeanne Quint. "Talking to Patients About Death." *Nursing Forum,* 9, no. 3:254-268, 1970. Also in *Contemporary Community Nursing*, edited by Barbara W. Spradely. Boston: Little, Brown and Company, 1975. Pp. 306-313.

Nurse expert identifies general cultural conditioning, personal and professional threat as factors making open talk about death difficult. Considers special problems created by cancer diagnosis. Describes cues patients give nurses about wanting to talk about death and offers suggestions for responses. Tells why attempting to make dying a personalized experience for patients is nursing challenge.

34. ______ . "The Concept of Care for a Child with Leukemia." *Nursing Forum*, 11, no. 2:194-204, 1972.

Discusses impact of diagnosis on child, his family, his caretakers. Identifies common maladaptive behavior patterns in such families. Distinguishes between cure and care concepts. Discusses ways to provide care that facilitates open communication, promotes child's participation in decisions affecting him, allows for expression of true feelings.

35. ______ . "Nursing Care for the Terminal Patients: A Psychosocial Approach," in *Psychosocial Aspects of Terminal Care*, pp. 145-151 (B-52).

Comments on definitional issues; identifies four types of nursing contacts with people facing death, noting ways nursing service needs vary accordingly. Says enunciated nursing goals of personalized care contrasts with reality of terminal nursing care situations. Cites research, clinical investigations. Discusses how systems-oriented approach can improve institutional care; ways nurses can influence, bring about change. Cites 62 references.

36. ______ . "Anticipatory Grief in Physicians and Nurses," in *Anticipatory Grief,* pp. 218-228 (B-53).

Comments on loss and grief in general and then focuses on professional loss and ways in which this kind of loss is responded to in the subcultures of nursing and medicine. Cites 20 references.

37. ______. "Death Influence in Clinical Practice: A Course Outline for the Nursing School Curriculum," in *The Nurse as Caregiver for the Terminal Patient and His Family,* pp. 227-243 (B-12).

Reprint of course outline used by author in course taught at University of Washington School of Nursing is offered as suggested model. Includes nine-page bibliography.

38. ______ . "Overview: Care, Cure, and the Challenge of Choice," in *The Nurse as Caregiver for the Terminal Patient and His Family,* pp. 9-30 (B-12).

Distinguishes between concepts of care and cure. Discusses problems dying and death pose for nurses. Includes comments on the impact of technology, the conflicting goals of practice, the non-accountability of psychosocial care, and depersonalized care practices. Elaborates on components of ethical practice, special problems precipitated by cancer. Comments on educational preparation of nurses needed for moving toward "goal of dignified and personalized care for each patient on his own terms." Cites 24 references.

39. BERGMAN, Abraham B. "Sudden Infant Death." *Nursing Outlook,* 20:775-777, December, 1972. Also in *Contemporary Nursing Series: Nursing of Children and Adolescents,* compiled by Andrea B. O'Connor. New York: American Journal of Nursing Company, 1975. Pp. 31-35.

Comments on syndrome, gives history, and discusses effect on parents who suffer guilt and anguish when not told death is unpredicatable and unpreventable.

40. BERGMAN, Abraham B., Margaret A. Pomeroy, and J. Bruce Beckwith. "The Psychiatric Toll of the Sudden Infant Death Syndrome." *General Practitioner,* 15:99-105, December, 1969. Available from National Foundation for Sudden Infant Death.

Gives factual information about the syndrome; notes false beliefs parents commonly hold. Discusses family's reaction to tragedy; uses letters from three mothers to describe anguish. Indicates how physician can be helpful.

41. BERMOSK, Loretta S. and Raymond J. Corsini, editors. *Critical Incidents in Nursing.* Philadelphia: W. B. Saunders Company, 1973. Selected pages. Entries A, B, C, and D listed below are four incidents taken from this publication in which 38 nurses present situations involving unresolved problems. Opinions and comments of consultants invited to react to and discuss the situations follow each incident.

A. "Dignity and Dying." Incident 19, pp. 160-170.

Patient/physician and physician/nurse conflict. Physician who refuses to inform questioning patient about her fatal prognosis becomes angered at nurse with opposite viewpoint who opens communication with patient shortly before patient's death. Reactions of seven consultants, including Jeanne Quint Benoliel, Avery Weisman.

B. "The Doctor Lets the Patient Die." Incident 14, pp. 127-133.

Forty-three-year-old cardiac patient tells both his own physician and emergency room nurse not to use heroic measures if heart stops. Patient arrests, nurse initiates resuscitation; patient arrests again and physician does not allow team to start resuscitation. Six discussants include Esther Hoffman and Avery Weisman.

C. "Helping the Patient Die." Incident 6, pp. 54-65.

In pact with dying woman, nurse gives patient triple dose of morphine to end her suffering. Jean Quint Benoliel and Avery Weisman are among nine discussants.

D. "A Last Request." Incident 21, pp. 179-186.

Patient asks nurse not to let wife see him die. Nurse honors request but action angers wife. Edwin S. Shneidman and Avery Weisman are among five who respond.

42. BINGER, C. M. and others. "Childhood Leukemia: Emotional Impact on Parent and Family." *New England Journal of Medicine,* 280:414-418, February, 1969.

Retrospective study of parents whose children died of leukemia reports initial reactions to diagnosis; children's awareness and parents' efforts to protect them; sources of support; benefits of mutual sharing; impact of child's dying and death on parents, siblings, grandparents; parents' suggestions for improving care.

43. BLEWETT, Laura J. "To Die at Home." *American Journal of Nursing,* 70:2602-2604, December, 1970. Also in *The Dying Patient: A Nursing Perspective,* pp. 264-267 (B-5).

Personal story of care given by four inactive nurses who make it possible for 39-year-old dying woman to remain at home with children and husband.

44. BLUMBERG, Jeanne E. and Eleanor E. Drummond. "Death, the Inevitable: An Approach," in *Nursing Care of the Long-Term Patient.*" New York: Springer Publishing Company, 1971. Pp. 107-124.

Discusses nursing care of dying patients in terms of observation, physical care, emotional care, treatment, teaching, counseling, economics. Clinical illustrations include student papers from "Death and the Curriculum," described in Entry A-84.

45. BONINE, Gladys N. "Students' Reactions to Children's Deaths." *American Journal of Nursing,* 67:1439-1440, July, 1967. Also in *The Dying Patient: A Nursing Perspective,* pp. 209-213 (B-6).

Instructor uses questionnaire and interview with 32 nursing students to learn how death of children affects the students. Gives sample student responses and suggestions for coping with dying and death of children.

46. BOZEMAN, Mary F., Charles E. Orbach, and Arthur M. Sutherland. "The Psychological Impact of Cancer and Its Treatment: III. The Adaptation of Mothers to the Threatened Loss of Their Children Through Leukemia: Part I." *Cancer,* 8, no. 1:1-19, 1955. Available from American Cancer Society. See Entry A-273 for Part II.

Study of mothers of 20 fatally ill children under age seven. Describes mothers' behavioral and emotional responses; their outpatient experiences; problems they encountered visiting hospitalized children; means they used for coping with impending loss; how they evaluated nurses; burdens of sibling's care, finances, travel. Explores ways mothers' needs were met through relationships with significant others; how children's parents supported each other.

47. BRAINARD, Franklin. "Rather than Scream." *Today's Health,* 49:32-37, June, 1971.

Fifty-one-year-old teacher-husband-father recounts experience of being told of fatal illness and what it means to live with threat of death. Says greatest need is for communication and sharing feelings.

48. BRAUER, Paul H. "Should the Patient Be Told the Truth?" *Nursing Outlook,* 8:672-676, December, 1960. Also in *Social Interaction and Patient Care,* edited by James K. Skipper and Robert C. Leonard. Philadelphia: J. B. Lippincott Company, 1965. Pp. 167-178.

Notes how scientific progress increases complexities involved in terminal illness. Stresses need to clarify terminology. Discusses impact of word "cancer" and how care, treatment are influenced by attitudes toward death. Explores truth-telling question and truth's relativity. Indicates need for careful assessment of patient's/family's understanding of disease and what honesty involves.

49. BRAVERMAN, Shirley J. "Death of a Monster." *American Journal of Nursing*, 69:1682-1683, August, 1969. Also in *The Dying Patient: A Nursing Perspective*, pp. 183-185 (B-6).

Young staff nurse describes personal reactions and distressed, conflicting feelings evoked in experience involving dying and death of a multiply deformed newborn admitted to pediatric ward.

50. BREUER, Judith. "Sharing a Tragedy." *American Journal of Nursing*, 76:758-759, May, 1976. Also in *Dying and Grief: Nursing Interventions,* pp. 162-164 (B-45).

Husband of nurse-patient is present during delivery, shares grief with wife when infant dies, but staff avoids contact with couple following infant's death.

51. BRIGHT, Florence and Sister M. Luciana France. "The Nurse and the Terminally Ill Child." *Nursing Outlook*, 15:39-42, September, 1967. Also in *The Dying Patient: A Nursing Perspective*, pp. 224-232 (B-6).

Describes work experiences at St. Jude Children's Research Hospital; its family-centered care philosophy that emphasizes normality; nursing interventions. Considers children's reactions to illness, incorporating research findings and own clinical observations.

52. BRIMIGION, Jeanne. "Living with Dying." *Nursing 72,* 2:23-27, June, 1972.

Nurse director of geriatric facility describes incident resulting in action that explored nurse's role in care of dying patients. Outlines activities undertaken to change attitudes of nurses "trained not to talk about dying or death."

53. BRUCE, Sylvia J. "Reactions of Nurses and Mothers to Stillbirths." *Nursing Outlook*, 10:88-91, February, 1962.

Discusses guilt and grief experienced with infant's loss; need for patients to express feelings, talk about loss. Illustrates helpful nurse actions and interactions.

54. del BUENO, Dorothy J. "We Didn't Know Better so We Did It Wrong." *RN Magazine*, 38:32-35+, October, 1975.

Tells of nonconstructive, rejecting behavior exhibited by nurses unable to accept a 34-year-old man's decision to die.

55. BUNCH, Barbara and Donna Zahra. "Dealing with Death: The Unlearned Role." *American Journal of Nursing*, 76:1486-1488, September, 1976. Also in *Dying and Grief: Nursing Interventions*, pp. 173-175 (B-45).

Notes that human behavior is learned. Suggestion that nurses can learn appropriate role behaviors for dying situations through role playing in groups is superficially presented.

56. BURKHALTER, Pamela. "Fostering Staff Sensitivity to the Dying Patient." *Supervisor Nurse*, 6:54-59, April, 1975.

Outlines means of promoting staff sensitivity through use of literature, clinical exercises, reaction diaries, role playing, films, and seminars. Comments on beneficial outcomes, potential problems.

57. BURNSIDE, Irene M. "You Will Cope of Course. . . . " *American Journal of Nursing*, 71:2354-2357, December, 1971. Also in *The Dying Patient: A Nursing Perspective*, pp. 117-122 (B-6).

Nurse describes reaction to diagnosis of husband's fatal illness and his 14 months of progressive deterioration; how this affected their children; how they coped after his death.

58. BUSCHMAN, Penelope R., Sarah L. Sheets, and Ann Wharton. "Use of Psychopharmacologic Agents in the Care of the Terminally Ill Child: A Nursing Overview," in *Psychopharmacologic Agents for the Terminally Ill and Bereaved*, pp. 287-290 (B-26).

Uses clinical examples in discussing how children's perception of pain differs from that of adults. Indicates effective care requires combination of medication and skilled nursing.

59. CAREY, Raymond G. "Living Until Death." *Hospital Progress*, 55:82-87, February, 1974. Also in *Death: The Final Stage of Growth*, pp. 75-86 (B-37).

Describes service and research program, involving 74 terminally ill persons, that attempted to determine factors for predicting who will cope best with dying and how helping professionals can make life more meaningful for dying patients.

60. CARLSON, Carolyn E. "Grief and Mourning," in *Behavioral Concepts and Nursing Intervention*, coordinated by Carolyn E. Carlson. Philadelphia: J. B. Lippincott Company, 1970. Pp. 95-115.

Provides examples to demonstrate that grief and mourning imply more than behavior related to death of loved ones. Defines terms, though clear distinctions not made in discussion. Comments on Engle's stages of grief and mourning and discusses nursing responsibilities and interventions in work with patients and families when death is expected.

61. CAROLINE, Nancy L. "Dying in Academe." *The New Physician*, 21:654-657, November, 1972. Available from Euthanasia Educational Council under title "Do Doctors Know the Real Enemy?"

Interaction between 78-year-old man ready to die and physician who fails to keep promise not to institute heroic measures. Patient found dead minus tubes and machine connections; scrawled note said, "Death is not the enemy, doctor. Inhumanity is."

62. CARPENTER, James O. and Charles M. Wylie. "On Aging, Dying, and Denying: Delivering Care to Older Dying Patients." *Public Health Reports*, 89, no. 5:403-407, 1974.

Notes greatest number of deaths occur within institutions, where focus upon cure weakens thrust for better care of dying aged and contributes to health care professional's denial of the significance of their care. Suggests social death contributes to biological death. Cites 15 references.

63. CARPENTER, Kathryn M. and J. Marion Stewart. "Parents Take Heart at City of Hope." *American Journal of Nursing*, 62:82-85, October, 1962.

Describes institutional facilities, staff composition. Tells of program encouraging parents to participate actively in care of their children with malignant tumors and leukemia and how this benefits children, parents, staff.

64. CARSON, Janice. "Learning from a Dying Patient." *American Journal of Nursing*, 71:333-334, February, 1971.

Senior nursing student describes her concerns, feelings, and responses in first experience with dying patient, a 44-year-old recent widow.

65. CAUGHILL, Rita E. "Coping with Death in Acute Care Units," in *The Dying Patient: A Supportive Approach*, pp. 95-123 (B-8).

Considers high death potential in emergency rooms, intensive and coronary care units, and patients' need for meaningful communication. Discusses problems related to: staff attitudes towards patient's family; coping with family's grief; notifying them of death; viewing body; providing emotional support. Describes enormous pressures nurses face; clinical examples illustrate how involvement with patients creates psychological stress. Discusses nurses' need for support; offers suggestions for helping staff members cope with the strong feelings their work evokes. Cites 17 references.

66. ______ . "Supportive Care and the Age of the Dying Patient," in *The Dying Patient: A Supportive Approach*, pp. 191-223 (B-8).

Explores attitudes toward death at different age levels; within this framework offers suggestions for nursing care of dying persons in early, middle, late adulthood. Gives clinical examples. Cites 36 references.

67. CHODOFF, Paul, Stanford B. Friedman, and David A. Hamburg. "Stress, Defenses, and Coping Behavior: Observations in Parents of Children with Malignant Disease." *American Journal of Psychiatry*, 120:743-749, February, 1964.

Reports that denial, isolation of affect, and motor activity were most common defenses used by 46 parents of 27 children participating in National Cancer Institute study. Notes ways denial was masked or projected; how anger and somatization were used. Discusses: usefulness of defenses in helping parents cope; influence of education, cultural background; manifestation and inhibition of anticipatory grief.

68. COMERFORD, Brenda. "Parental Anticipatory Grief and Guidelines for Caregivers," in *Anticipatory Grief*, pp. 147-157 (B-53).

A mother's poignant story of a family's loving care of and open communication with an aware dying child during the 18-month period preceding her death at age six. Offers 43 suggestions "to guide both physicians and parents during the course of a child's terminal illness."

69. CORDER, Michael P. and Robert L. Anders. "Death and Dying – Oncology Discussion Group." *Journal of Psychiatric Nursing and Mental Health Services*, 12:11-14, July/August, 1974.

Nurse and physician report sketchily on groups and their benefit to patients and staff at Lettermann Army Medical Center.

70. COTTER, Sister Zita. "Institutional Care of the Terminally Ill." *Hospital Progress*, 52:43-48, June, 1971.

Believes effective care of dying patients requires "a community of caring persons, and considers St. Christopher's Hospice an ideal model. Enumerates ways in which caring is evidenced and respect for human dignity is conveyed.

71. ______ . "On Not Getting Better." *Hospital Progress*, 56:60-73, March, 1972.

Says use of phrase in title often indicates a patient's awareness of approaching death. Sample interactions demonstrate beginning awareness, need for delicate listening and responding to establish climate of openness. Gives two basic ground rules for interacting with dying patients.

72. COYNE, A. Barbara. "The Nurse's Responsibilities," in *The Nurse as Caregiver for the Terminal Patient and His Family*, pp. 66-73 (B-12).

Says nurses must assume responsibility for helping their fatally ill clients live until they die and for helping families repattern their relationships and activities. Presents illustrative case report.

73. CRAVEN, Joan and Florence S. Wald. "Hospice Care for Dying Patients." *American Journal of Nursing*, 75:1816-1822, October, 1975. Also in *Dying and Grief: Nursing Interventions*, pp. 21-33 (B-45).

Comments on hospice movement and on projected Connecticut hospice. Discusses management of distressing disease symptoms, ways of controlling chronic pain, getting patient/family actively involved in patient's care, use of interdisciplinary team in care program.

74. CRAYTOR, Josephine K. "Talking with Persons Who Have Cancer." *American Journal of Nursing*, 69:744-748, April, 1969. Also in *Nursing and the Cancer Patient*, pp. 92-99 (B-7).

Says "Cancer is still a dread disease to patients, nurses, and physicians." Says conversing with cancer patients risks "discussion of pain, death, loss . . . ." Examples of nurse-patient interactions illustrate listening, feedback, and giving information.

75. DAVIDOFF, Leo M. "What One Neurosurgeon Does," in *Should the Patient Know the Truth*? pp. 88-92 (B-58).

Stresses that what patients are told about their condition should depend on the type of person they are; that the way patient asks and how patient is told are important.

76. DAVIDSON, Ramona P. "Let's Talk About Death: To Give Care in Terminal Illness." *American Journal of Nursing*, 66: 74-75, January, 1966. Also in *The Dying Patient: A Nursing Perspective*, pp. 78-81 (B-6).

Describes two patients who stimulated nurses to improve care of dying patients. Comments briefly on five other patients from whom nurses learned that the most common needs are for physical comfort and communication.

77. DAVIS, Barbara. ". . . Until Death Ensues." *Nursing Clinics of North America*, 7:303-309, June, 1972.

Interviews with 54 nursing-home patients indicate their need to talk about death and dying. Suggests ways to assist patient's family/significant others to prepare for his death; lists concepts for formulating and implementing nursing care plans for dying patients.

78. "Death in the First Person." *American Journal of Nursing*, 70:336, February, 1970. Also in *The Dying Patient: A Nursing Perspective*, pp. 181-182 (B-5). Also in *Death: The Final Stage of Growth*, pp. 25-26 (B-37).

Dying nursing student shares feelings about her situation; pleads for more personalized care from care providers.

79. DIAZ, Elizabeth. "A Death on the Pediatric Ward." *Hospital topics*, 47:83-87, May, 1969.

Child-care worker involved in long-term care of a child on pediatric unit describes impact of last hours of child's life on herself and others; how children on the unit were informed of child's death.

80. DOBROF, Rose. "Community Resources and Care of the Terminally Ill and Their Families," in *Psychosocial Aspects of Terminal Care*, pp. 290-306 (B-52).

Social worker relates stories of mother who attempted to kill her doomed baby when she could no longer care for it and of post-stroke patient of 79 discharged from hospital to care of ill, 81-year-old husband. Uses these and other stories to illustrate ways institutions fail people and add to their suffering. Suggests action to promote effective care since lack of resources not major reason needed services were not provided in cases cited.

81. DOVENMUEHLE, Robert H. "Affective Responses to Life-Threatening Cardiovascular Disease," in *Death and Dying: Attitudes of Patient and Doctor*. Group for the Advancement of Psychiatry. Symposium No. 11. New York: Group for the Advancement of Psychiatry, 1965. Pp. 607-613.

Comments on interpersonal and other factors that influence patients' behavior; cultural pressures that influence patients and physicians in life-threatening illness; approaches to dying patients.

82. DOWNEY, Gregg W. "Dying Patients Still Have Human Needs." *Modern Hospital*, 114:78-81, March, 1970.

Summarizes University of Chicago seminar on dying patients where family dynamics expert related benefits of joint patient/family interviews, nurse expert described nurse responses to dying patients, and Kubler-Ross told of work with dying and interviewed a patient before the group.

83. DRUMMOND, Eleanor E. "Communication and Comfort for the Dying Patient." *Nursing Clinics of North America*, 5:55-63, March, 1970.

Describes situations promoting and blocking communication. Comments on patient's right to know; use of denial/avoidance; providing spiritual comfort; benefits of physical comforts; importance of maintaining pain relief while keeping patients alert. Argues against heroic measures.

84. DRUMMOND, Eleanor E. and Jeanne E. Blumberg. "Death and the Curriculum: How We Discuss Death in the Adult Course for Registered Nurse Students." *Journal of Nursing Education*, 1:21-28, May/June, 1962.

Nurse-teachers provide death-related content upon students' request for help. Excerpts from students' papers illustrate specific concepts; three reprinted papers recount students' feelings and reactions in personal experiences with dying patients.

85. DUBREY, Rita J. and Laura A. Terrill. "Loneliness of the Dying Person." *Omega*, 6, no. 4:357-371, 1974.

Report of interview study conducted by nurses involving 50 terminally ill hospitalized patients. Feelings of loneliness, nature of important relationships, and effect of cancer on life of each patient explored. Findings in agreement with other research that "terminally ill patients will talk about their concerns if someone will sit and listen." Alludes to implications for nursing care.

86. "The Dying Person's Bill of Rights." *American Journal of Nursing*, 75:99, January, 1975.

Sixteen first-person statements developed by inservice education workshop participants.

87. EASSON, William M. "Care of the Young Patient Who Is Dying." *Journal of the American Medical Association*, 205:203-207, July 22, 1968.

Discusses usual reactions to death in child, adolescent, and young adult; notes how normal age-appropriate emotional responses complicate therapeutic management. Considers treatment for each group; behavior exhibited by parents, family in process of mourning.

88. ______ . "The Family of the Dying Child." *Pediatric Clinics of North America*, 19:1157-1165, November, 1972.

Physician discusses rationale for telling parents jointly about child's fatal illness and for follow-up conferences; considers mourning behaviors, consequences of family completing mourning before child's death, maintaining involvement, reactions to child's death.

89. EATON, James S. Jr. "Coping with Staff Grief," in *The Nurse as Caregiver for the Terminal Patient and His Family*, pp. 140-146 (B-12).

Believes nurses and physicians rarely recognize their mutual responsibility for providing an emotionally supportive environment which deals with the needs of dying patients as well as recognizing, dealing with, and accepting their own emotional needs when faced with the loss of a patient. Pleads for professionals to support one another, especially at times of stress involving dying and death.

90. EISMAN, Roberta. "Why Did Joc Die?" *American Journal of Nursing*, 71:501-503, March, 1971. Also in *The Dying Patient: A Nursing Perspective*, pp. 56-60 (B-6).

Nurse describes care provided 65-year-old man on research unit and changes in his behavior when transferred to unfamiliar conventional unit where staff viewed patient's condition as hopeless and where he died within two weeks.

91. ELDER, Ruth G. "Dying in the U.S.A." *International Journal of Nursing Studies*, 10:171-184, August, 1973. Also in *Nursing Digest*, 2:2-11, May, 1974. Also in *Nursing Digest: 1975 Focus on Care of the Elderly*, pp. 61-70; *Nursing Digest: 1975, Review of Medicine and Surgery,* pp. 108-117; *Nursing Digest: 1975 Review of Psychiatry and Mental Health*, pp. 108-117. Wakefield, Mass.: Contemporary Publishing, 1975.

Reports changes in life expectancy, family structure/function and their consequences in relation to dying and death. Cites literature and research in comments on death and dying attitudes, question of truth telling, concepts of awareness contexts, dying trajectories, and nonaccountability. Suggests care for dying is part of larger problem, broader issue of depersonalization associated with organizational bureaucracy. Cites 44 references (none in *Nursing Digest* reprints).

92. ______ . "Dying and Society," in *The Dying Patient: A Supportive Approach*, pp. 1-29 (B-8).

Revision of "Dying in the U.S.A." cited in Entry A-91.

93. ELKINTON, Russell J. "When Do We Let the Patient Die?" *Annals of Internal Medicine*, 68:695-700, March, 1968.

Says physician must cope with decisions about dying patients involving life prolongation, use of ordinary or extraordinary measures, definitions of death *now*, regardless of moral or philosophical decisions society may make in future. Discusses decisions affecting patients with different diagnoses.

94. ELMORE, James L. and Adriaan Verwoerdt. "Psychological Reactions to Impending Death." *Hospital Topics*, 45:35-36, November, 1967.

Results of study involving 30 fatally ill patients indicate their feelings of hopelessness and "constriction" of future becomes greater near death. Discusses: use of therapeutic regression; implications for care; daily care plans that emphasize satisfaction from small accomplishments.

95. ENGEL, George L. "Grief and Grieving." *American Journal of Nursing;* 64:93-98, September, 1964. Also in *Psychiatric Nursing: A Book of Readings*, second edition, edited by Dorothy Mereness. Dubuque, Iowa: William C. Brown Company, Publishers, 1970, pp. 2-12. Also in *The Psychodynamics of Patient Care* by Lawrence H. Schwartz and Jane L. Schwartz. Englewood Cliffs, N.J.: Prentice-Hall, 1972, pp. 376-387. Also in *The Dying Patient: A Nursing Perspective*, pp. 105-116 (B-6).

Describes and discusses sequences of events characterizing normal grief; steps necessary for resolving loss; process of idealization; factors influencing outcome of mourning work. Eight recommendations for nursing action in situations involving dying and death of patients.

96. EVANS, Audrey E. and S. Edin. "If a Child Must Die. . . ." *New England Journal of Medicine*, 278:138-142, January 18, 1968.

Gives rationale for care approach when focus is on shielding child from knowledge of his dying and protecting him from death fears. Outlines care measures found in each of three identified stages of dying roughly determined by course of disease.

97. EVANS, Dale F. and Gail Sutton. "A Case for Consultation." *Nursing Clinics of North America*, 8:751-756, December, 1973.

Describes problems created by hospital staff's involvement with dying patient and his wife and outcomes of nursing consultation experience that assisted nursing personnel in helping patient and family to cope with impending death.

98. "Experiences with Dying Patients." *American Journal of Nursing*, 73:1058-1064, June, 1973. A special feature. Starred

(*) titles also in *Dying and Grief: Nursing Interventions*, pp. 51-52; 52-53 (B-45).

Eight nurses give brief personal accounts of memorable experiences with dying patients. Stories are titled: A Boy Who Couldn't Talk; Some Patients Prefer Silence; Won't Someone Care?; *It's Hard to Sit with Death: *When the Hour Comes; The Search for Meaning; It Only Takes a Little Time to Listen; Listening to Those Who Can Speak and Those Who Cannot.

99. FEDER, Samuel L. "Attitudes of Patients with Advanced Malignancy," in *Death and Dying: Attitudes of Patient and Doctor.* Group for the Advancement of Psychiatry. Symposium No. 11. New York: Group for the Advancement of Psychiatry, 1965. Pp. 614-622. Also in *Death: Current Perspectives,* pp. 430-438 (B-56).

Observations of 100 patients with malignant disease indicate almost all knew they had malignancy and that their greatest concern was progressive isolation. Discusses importance of communication and need to focus on problems of living.

100. FEIFEL, Herman. "The Function of Attitudes Toward Death," in *Death and Dying: Attitudes of Patient and Doctor*. Group for the Advancement of Psychiatry. Symposium No. 11. New York: Group for the Advancement of Psychiatry, 1965. Pp. 632-641.

Author discusses own research and physicians' resistance to his study of seriously and terminally ill patients. Cites studies comparing opinions of patient and physician about telling patient he is dying. Supports telling, with emphasis on how done.

101. FEIGENBERG, Loma. "Care and Understanding of the Dying: A Patient-Centered Approach." *Omega*, 6, no. 2:81-94, 1975

Psychiatrist, former radiologist, describes psychotherapy approach of focussing exclusively on dying patient, with therapist making no contact with patient's significant others after therapy begins. Visits that occurred weekly during initial terminal stage of illness are increased and become less formal as disease progresses and condition deteriorates, requiring therapist to be on constant call in the final stage.

102. FLEMING, Ruth P. "Good Physical Care, Priority for the Dying." *RN Magazine*, 37:46+, April, 1974.

Nurse cites examples of physical nursing care activities that enhance patients' well-being with reminder that physical and psychological care are interdependent.

103. FLETCHER, George P. "Prolonging Life: Some Legal Considerations," in *Euthanasia and the Right to Death*, edited by A. B. Downing. New York: Humanities Press, 1970. Pp. 71-84. Also in *Death: Current Perspectives*, pp. 484-497 (B-56).

Comments on medical and legal problems created by new medical techniques for prolonging life. Expounds on legal intricacies involved in answering the question, "Is the physician's discontinuing aid to a terminal patient an act or omission?" Concludes that physicians "are in a position to fashion their own law to deal with cases of prolongation of life."

104. FLETCHER, Joseph. "Ethics and Euthanasia." *American Journal of Nursing*, 73:670-675, April, 1973. Also in *Dying and Grief: Nursing Interventions*, pp. 65-73 (B-45).

Discusses need for code of ethics based on quality of life and for life/death definitions in keeping with new realities. Argues clinical decisions in hospitals frequently prolong dying rather than living. Defines and discusses four kinds of euthanasia. Believes real issue is moral justification of suicide, mercy killing. Advocates active euthanasia. See Weber, Entry A-367, for opposing view.

105. FOLLETT, Elvie. "No Time for Fear." *The Canadian Nurse*, 66:30-40, January, 1970.

Nurse instructor tells about courageous 15-year-old dying boy and positive effect he had on all who knew him.

106. FOND, Karen I. "Dealing with Death and Dying Through Family-Centered Care." *The Nursing Clinics of North America*, 7:53-64, March, 1972.

Considers essentials of care plan for fatally ill child; meaning of loss for those involved; how attitudes toward death influence care; ways of facilitating parent participation and consideration of dying child's siblings; importance of understanding grieving process and stages of dying. Uses examples to illustrate concepts.

107. FORD, J. Massynberde. "Living with Death," in *ANA Clinical Sessions: American Nurses' Association, 1974 San Francisco*. New York: Appleton-Century-Crofts, 1975. Pp. 221-230.

Former nurse, now a scripture scholar, compares ways of dying in the United States and England; shows Kubler-Ross's stages of dying are reflected in Biblical writings; focuses upon and shares personal experiences of having faced death three times.

108. FOX, Jean E. "Reflections on Cancer Nursing." *American Journal of Nursing*, 66:1317-1319, June, 1966. Also in *Nursing and the Cancer Patient*, pp. 100-105 (B-7).

Identifies three stages of care; focuses on terminal stage of disease when aim is to enable patient to die well. Describes nursing care of 30-year-old mother of three from announcement of fatal prognosis to leave taking of children and death.

109. FREDLUND, Delphie J. "A Nurse Looks at Children's Questions About Death," in *ANA Clinical Sessions: American Nurses' Association, 1970 Miami*. New York: Appleton-Centry-Crofts, 1971. Pp. 105-112.

Discusses findings of study involving four-year-olds and interviews with mothers regarding children's ideas, feelings, knowledge of death. Enumerates nursing implications.

110. FRENCH, Jean and Doris R. Schwartz. "Terminal Care at Home in Two Cultures." *American Journal of Nursing*, 73: 502-505, March, 1973.

Public health nurses discuss ways cultures of Navajo woman dying of cancer and Italian-born man with organic brain disease influenced nursing care given and accepted by patients and families who rejected hospitalization.

111. FRIEDMAN, Stanford B. and others. "Behavioral Observations on Parents Anticipating the Death of a Child." *Pediatrics*, 32:610-625, October, 1963.

Elaboration of the Chordoff, Friedman, Hamburg study cited in Entry A-67.

112. FULTON, Robert and Julie Fulton. "A Psychosocial Aspect of Terminal Care: Anticipatory Grief." *Omega*, 2:91-100, May, 1971. Also in *Death and Identity*, pp. 323-335 (B-21).

Discusses growing trend for dying and death to take place in institutions and effects of this upon patients and their families. Distinguishes between "high-grief-potential" and "low-grief-potential" deaths. Discusses anticipatory grief, citing studies illustrating ways it influences behavior and creates problems for dying patient and family. Suggests ways professionals can be more helpful. Cites 18 references. See Entry C-36 for audio-cassette information.

113. ______ . "Anticipatory Grief: A Psychosocial Aspect of Terminal Care," in *Psychosocial Aspects of Terminal Care,* pp. 227-242 (B-52).

Content identical to "A Psychosocial Aspect of Terminal Care: Anticipatory Grief" cited in Entry A-112 except footnote and reference formats differ.

114. FULTON, Robert and Phyllis A. Langton. "Attitudes Toward Death: An Emerging Mental Health Problem." *Nursing Forum*, 3, no. 1: 104-112, 1964.

Discusses shift from traditional religious beliefs about death to secular orientation and general reluctance of both health care professionals and laity to deal with dying and death. Indicates how hospital staffs' attitudes and beliefs affect their behavior toward the dying and death of patients.

115. FUTTERMAN, Edward H., Irwin Hoffman, and Melvin Sabshin. "Parental Anticipatory Mourning," in *Psychosocial Aspects of Terminal Care*, pp. 243-272 (B-52).

Data from study of 23 sets of parents with children dying of leukemia suggests emergence of a five-part sequential process of anticipatory mourning. Discusses these processes and their significance; illustrates points with excerpts from parents' comments. Cites 37 references.

116. GARTNER, Claudine R. "Growing Up to Dying: The Child, the Parents, and the Nurse," in *The Dying Patient: A Supportive Approach*, pp. 159-190 (B-8).

Considers developmental tasks of infant, toddler, preschool/school-age child, adolescent; indicates similarities and differences of a dying child's needs in each period. Offers concrete suggestions for care of dying infants, more generalized suggestions for care in other age periods. Comments on sudden infant death syndrome; parents' reactions to child's impending death.

117. GEIS, Dorothy P. "Mothers' Perceptions of Care Given Their Dying Children." *American Journal of Nursing*, 65:105-107, February, 1965. Also in *The Dying Patient: A Nursing Perspective*, pp. 238-245 (B-6).

Twenty-six mothers of children who died were interviewed, shared impressions of care nurses gave. Focus was on helpful and hurtful relationships, not physical or technical care. Suggestions for improving care centered on interpersonal relationships.

118. GELEIN, Janet L. "Needs of the Terminally Ill Aged," in *ANA Clinical Sessions: American Nurses' Association, 1972 Detroit*. New York: Appleton-Century-Crofts, 1973. Pp. 39-44.

Refers to universal needs of aging identified by Simmons, Maslow's hierarchy of needs, and gerontological life style theory; alludes to implications of these for nursing the dying. Cites 24 references.

119. GESSNER, Barbara A. "The Health Care Team and Planning for the Patient," in *Oral Care of the Aging and Dying Patient*, edited by Austin H. Kutscher and Ivan K. Goldberg. Springfield, Ill.: Charles C Thomas, Publisher, 1973. Pp. 144-153.

Nurse discusses the physiological and psychological aspects of care for patients with cancer of the head and neck. Focuses on the oral cavity and the need for and significance of communication between patient and care-giving personnel.

120. GLASER, Barney G. and Anselm L. Strauss. "The Social Loss of Dying Patients." *American Journal of Nursing*, 64:119-121, June, 1964. Also in *The Dying Patient: A Nursing Perspective*, pp. 141-147 (B-6).

Discusses how the social value of a patient influences impact his dying and death have on nurse and care he receives, how social loss is calculated. Says alertness to social values staff bring to hospital also is pertinent.

121. ______ . "Dying on Time: Arranging the Final Hours of Life in a Hospital." *Transaction Social Science and Modern Society*, 2:27-31, May/June 1965. Also in *Confrontations of Death*, pp. 104-108 (B-54).

Describes ways nurses try to establish expectations regarding certainty and time of death and how expectation or nonexpectation of death affects nurse behavior and composure. Comments on advantages of open awareness, care complexities in other awareness states.

122. ______ . "Dying in Hospitals," in *Chronic Illness and the Quality of Life*, by Anselm L. Strauss. St. Louis: The C. V. Mosby Company, 1975. Pp. 119-129.
Excerpts from Chapter Eight of *Time for Dying* (Entry B-24). Considers issues underlying and factors influencing decisions of patient and family in determining whether death will occur at home or in hospital.

123. GLASER, Robert J. "Innovations and Heroic Acts in Prolonging Life," in *The Dying Patient*, pp. 102-128 (B-5).
Considers moral, ethical, social, and legal problems created by ability to prolong, extend life. Comments on rise of organ transplants; need for redefinition of death and criteria for life prolongation and termination; problems of organ supply/demand; cost of heroics; quality of prolonged life.

124. GOLDBERG, Stanley B. "Family Tasks and Reactions in the Crisis of Death." *Social Casework*, 54:389-405, July, 1973. Also in *Nursing Digest*, 2:21-26, May, 1974. Also in *Nursing Digest: 1975 Review of Maternal Child Health*. Wakefield, Mass.: Contemporary Publishing, 1975. Pp. 118-123.
Discusses death as an unanticipated crisis with focus on family readjustment tasks rather than on individual mourning tasks. Considers role reorganization, increased solidarity, object replacement.

125. GOLDFOGEL, Lenda. "Working with the Parent of a Dying Child." *American Journal of Nursing*, 70:1675-1679, August, 1970. Also in *The Dying Patient: A Nursing Perspective*, pp. 123-133 (B-6).
Nurse involved in care of terminally ill six-year-old describes efforts to help mother adapt to his illness and anticipated death; comments on feelings and coping behaviors of self, child, mother.

126. GOLDIN, Phyllis S. "No Second Chance." *American Journal of Nursing*, 72:478-479, March, 1972.
Senior nursing student reports feelings about and reactions to emergency room experience where she witnessed a man's sudden death, activities of staff, grief of his family.

127. GOLDSTEIN, Eda G. and Sidney Malitz. "Psychotherapy and Pharmacotherapy as Enablers in the Anticipatory Grief of a Dying Patient: A Case Study," in *Anticipatory Grief*, pp. 285-295 (B-53).

Social worker and physician analyst, collaborating in treatment of psychiatric patient with aim of helping this 36-year-old woman to live a fuller life, continue to work with her after discovery of malignant condition, with goal of helping her to die.

128. GONDA, Thomas A. "Pain and Addiction in Terminal Illness," in *Loss and Grief*, pp. 261-269 (B-51).

Distinguishes between pain at personal and interpersonal levels; discusses complex interweaving of pain determinants on neurophysiological, psychophysiological, sociopsychological levels. Comments on physicians' reluctance to increase drug dosages; alternatives in managing pain behavior.

129. GOOGE, Mary C. "The Death of a Young Man." *American Journal of Nursing*, 64:133-135, November, 1964.

Nursing student describes her involvement in nursing care of dying 17-year-old boy – her first encounter with dying patient.

130. GORTNER, Susan R. "Death with Dignity: Ethical Issues in the Proposed Legislation," in *ANA Clinical Sessions: American Nurses' Association, 1974 San Francisco*. New York: Appleton-Century-Crofts, 1975. Pp. 169-176.

Sees concept of euthanasia central to issue. Comments on informed consent; right to refuse medical treatment; physician's views and practice; alternatives to legislation. Includes two samples of living wills. Cites 23 references.

131. GOTTHEIL, Edward, Wealtha C. McGurn, and Otto Pollak. "Is It Right to Joke with a Dying Man?" *Prism*, 2:16-21, December, 1974. Reprinted as "Truth and/or Hope for the Dying Patient" in *Nursing Digest*, 4:12-14, March/April,1976.

Comments on rationale for telling patients of impending death and questions supposed benefits of this knowledge. Discusses denial process and potential deleterious effects of interfering with it. Speculates whether knowledge of fatal prognosis interferes with will to live.

132. GREEN, Morris. "Care of the Dying Child." *Pediatrics*, 40:492-497, Part 2, September, 1967.

Condensation and rearrangement of the Solnit and Green article cited in Entry A-337, plus comment on management principles.

133. GREEN-EPNER, Carol S. "The Dying Child," in *The Dying Patient: A Supportive Approach*, pp. 125-157 (B-8).

Discusses how the death taboo in current American culture creates additional problems for dying child; concepts of death in both healthy and ill children; major psychological needs of dying child. Defines play; distinguishes between play therapy and the therapeutic play that nurses can use "as a means of communication and emotional release" for dying child. Cites 57 references.

134. GREENLEAF, Nancy P. "Stereotyped Sex-role Ranking of Caregivers and Quality Care for Dying Patients," in *The Nurse as Caregiver for the Terminal Patient and His Family*, pp. 185-193 (B-12).

Focuses on the interpersonal crises unexpected death of a hospitalized patient precipitates in caregivers, how it affects their shared experience, their humanity, and ability to give care. Suggests stereotyped roles of nurse and physician create barriers, reduce possibilities for sharing experiences or providing mutual support and comfort.

135. GRIFFIN, Jerry J. "Family Decision: A Crucial Factor in Terminating Life." *American Journal of Nursing*, 75:795-796, May, 1975. Also in *Dying and Grief: Nursing Interventions*, pp. 84-47 (B-45).

Clergyman describes need for time and readiness of all significant persons involved in reaching decision to permit action for removal of mechanical life support measures from a loved one.

136. GROLLMAN, Earl A. "Prologue: Explaining Death to Children," in *Explaining Death to Children*, pp. 3-37 (B-27).

Comments on fear of death as cultural and human phenomenon; how children can understand meaning of death; what parents should and should not say about death; ways children experience grief; how to help children who lose a loved one.

137. GUIMOND, Joyce. "We Knew Our Child Was Dying." *American Journal of Nursing*, 74:248-249, February, 1974.

Complications from mumps results in tragedy for parents of an eight-year-old boy; their anguish is compounded by false cheer and social tone of hospital staff with whom they interact.

138. GYULAY, Jo-Eileen. "Interactions and Reactions of Terminally Ill Children and Their Parents," in *ANA Clinical Sessions: American Nurses' Association, 1974 San Francisco.* New York: Appleton-Century-Crofts, 1975. Pp. 92-98.

Advocates openness and honesty between dying children and adult caretakers, especially parents; illustrates how child's behavior and communications are affected by parents; offers examples of nursing interaction for facilitating dying child's care.

139. ______ . "The Forgotten Grievers." *American Journal of Nursing,* 75:1476-1479, September, 1975. Also in *Dying and Grief: Nursing Interventions,* pp. 128-135 (B-45).

Discusses withdrawal or exclusion of fathers from participation in dying child's care; how dying situation evokes fathers' anger, guilt, other feelings. Notes impact of dying and death on siblings, grandparents, others knowing or involved with child.

140. ______ . "Care of the Dying Child." *Nursing Clinics of North America,* 11:95-107, March, 1976. Available from American Cancer Society.

Focuses on nursing care involved in terminal phase of fatal illness considering briefly: child's state of awareness/consciousness; family needs and family's participation in physical care; considerations related to vital sign monitoring, equipment, respiratory problems, seizure and temperature control, physical appearance, control of pain, rest/sleep, eating patterns, nutritional needs.

141. HACKETT, Thomas P. "How to Help the Dying Patient." *Medical Economics,* 43:148-149+, June, 1966.

Considers conspiracy of silence a major problem in care management. Cites arguments for not telling patient his condition. Notes subtle ways patients ask for truth. Gives clinical examples of benefits derived from open communication.

142. HACKETT, Thomas P. and Avery D. Weisman. "The Treatment of the Dying," in *Current Psychiatric Therapies,* Volume 2, edited by Jules H. Masserman. New York: Grune and Sratton, 1962. Pp. 121-126.

Reports on work with terminally ill patients. Comments on middle knowledge, denial by patients and physicians, consequences of nondisclosure, communication needs of dying patients, the many faces of truth, feelings of helplessness physicians experience.

143. ______ . "Reactions to the Imminence of Death," in *The Threat of Impending Disaster: Contributions to the Psychology of Stress*, edited by George H. Grosse, Henry Wechsler, and Milton Greenblatt. Cambridge, Mass.: The M. I. T. Press, 1964. Pp. 300-311.

Reports ways patients with terminal cancer facing certain death and patients with severe cardiac disease facing imminent death react to threat and employ denial in coping with their situation. Discusses ways interpersonal relationships influencing middle knowledge differ with each group.

144. ______ . "Denial as a Factor in Patients with Heart Disease and Cancer." *Annals of the New York Academy of Sciences,* 164:802-817, 1969.

Report of study comparing 20 patients from each group; exploration of relation between life-threatening illness and denial revealed patients have similar responses to threat of death despite treatment differences; cancer patients expressed greater concern about symptom control. Comprises Chapter Six of *On Dying and Denying* (Entry B-66).

145. HAGAN, Joan M. "Infant Death: Nursing Interaction and Intervention with Grieving Families." *Nursing Forum*, 13, no. 4: 371-385, 1974.

Public health nurse reports findings, describes activities, and indicates value of "death visiting" to families following infant's death. Discusses impact on mother and rest of family.

146. HAMPE, Sandra O. "Needs of the Grieving Spouse in a Hospital Setting." *Nursing Research*, 24:113-120, March/April, 1975. Also in *Dying and Grief: Nursing Interventions*, pp. 100-117 (B-45).

Report of interviews with 27 spouses of dying patients attempting to have them identify their needs and the ways in which nurses were helpful to them. Nurse seen as helping dying mate rather than interviewed spouse.

147. HANCOCK, Shiela. "Care of the Dying. A Death in the Family: A Lay View." *British Medical Journal*, 1:29-30, January 6, 1973.

Author tells of impact on learning of mother's fatal prognosis. Describes minimum assistance from health care personnel during her dying. Contrasts with care provided her dying husband and support given self at St. Christopher's Hospice.

148. [Hanlan, Archie J.] "Notes of a Dying Professor." *The Pennsylvania Gazette*, 60:18-24, March, 1972. Also in *Nursing Outlook*, 20:502-506, August, 1972. Also in *Nursing Digest*, 2:36-42, May, 1974.

Tells of traumas experienced during hospitalization for diagnosis. Describes evasive physician responses; depersonalized care; personnel's actions and comments that generated anxiety, fear, confusion; impact of fatal prognosis announced hour before discharge.

149. HARDGROVE, Carol and Louise H. Warrick. "How Shall We Tell the Children?" *American Journal of Nursing*, 74:448-450, March, 1974. Also in *Dying and Grief: Nursing Interventions*, pp. 156-161 (B-45).

Suggestions and guidelines to assist parents in telling their children about death of an expected baby.

150. HAY, Donald and Donald Oken. "The Psychological Stresses of Intensive Care Unit Nursing." *Psychosomatic Medicine*, 34: 109-118, March/April, 1972.

Dramatic description – based on interviews, informal contacts, and work of one physician as nursing staff member – of work setting that repeatedly exposes nurse to dying patients and death. Examines situational, psychological, interpersonal, administrative factors, and the complex adaptive maneuvers they evoke.

151. HAYS, Joyce S. "The Night Neil Died." *Nursing Outlook*, 10:801-803, December, 1962.

Categorizes and comments briefly on responses elicited from nurses who described their feelings and behavior upon death of 10-year-old patient.

152. HEINEMANN, Henry O. "Human Values in the Medical Care of the Terminally Ill," in *Psychosocial Aspects of Terminal Care*, pp. 19-30 (B-52).

Asks why needs of dying patients are not met by facilities in society; whether deficiencies reflect general attitudes or health professionals' lack of training. Comments on ethical issues, dilemmas created by advancing technology, disregard for consequences of some medical innovations, problems in providing terminal care.

153. HENDERSON, Edward. "The Approach to the Patient with an Incurable Disease," in *Psychosocial Aspects of Terminal Care*, pp. 57-61 (B-52).

Believes preserving "integrity of the patient's concept of himself" must be paramount concern in care of the dying. Uses patient histories to illustrate how negative or positive attitudes and behaviors of family and friends influenced responses of patients with leukemia.

154. HENDRICKSON, Sharon. "A Philosophy of Death Made Personal." *American Journal of Nursing*, 76:90, January, 1976. Dying nurse shares feelings about her impending death.

155. HERSHEY, Nathan. "The Law and the Nurse: On the Question of Prolonging Life." *American Journal of Nursing*, 71: 521-522, March, 1971.

Notes nurses' involvement in decisions to prolong or end life; says legal approach can help, although concepts of meaningful life increase decision complexities and decisions to start heroic measures differ from decisions to stop those started.

156. HERTER, Fredric P. "The Right to Die with Dignity," in *Death and Bereavement*, edited by Austin H. Kutscher. Springfield, Ill.: Charles C Thomas Publishers, 1969. Pp. 14-19.

Expresses value of sharing reality of situation with dying person and need to prepare for death in practical, spiritual, emotional ways. Describes family situation that illustrates positive effects of sharing.

157. HERTZBERG, Leonard J. "Cancer and the Dying Patient." *American Journal of Psychiatry*, 128:806-814, January, 1972.

Psychiatrist describes cancer research unit and patients' reactions to cancer and unit. Discusses interventions used and work with staff to foster more effective relationships with patients. Considers family involvement crucial.

158. HEUSINKVELD, Karen B. "Cues to Communication with the Terminal Cancer Patient." *Nursing Forum*, 11, no. 1:105-113, 1972.

Believing denial a useful defense for promoting patient comfort, nurse clinician describes work with dying patients in effort to determine its effectiveness.

159. HEYMANN, David A. "Discussions Meet Needs of Dying Patients." *Hospitals*, 48:57-58+, July 16, 1974.

Tells of first group meeting; development of guidelines; how meetings aided staff at Veteran's Hospital to meet patients' psychosocial needs and to learn more about dying and death.

160. HINTON, John. "The Physical and Mental Distress of the Dying." *Quarterly Journal of Medicine*, 23:1-21, January, 1963.

Reports study comparing physical discomforts, mental states, and personal life history of 102 dying hospitalized patients with 102 patients suffering serious, nonfatal disease. Data indicate greater intensity or incidence of unrelieved physical distress, depression, anxiety in dying group. Three out of four physically suffering patients were aware of dying. Describes study methodology. Includes tables, histograms; gives five-page discussion on results.

161. ______ . "The Dying and the Doctor," in *Man's Concern with Death*, pp. 36-45 (B-63).

Believes those with fatal illness usually suspect they are dying but frequently deceive themselves about recovery, and that their physicians encourage pretense. Discusses advantages and hazards inherent in pretense, reticence of physicians to deal openly with patients, use of avoidance tactics, patient reaction and response to open acknowledgment of prognosis.

162. ______ . "Assessing the Views of the Dying." *Social Science and Medicine*, 5:37-43, February, 1971.

Discusses difficulties in exploring attitudes and needs of persons with terminal illness: when interviewers use techniques allowing patients to express their views and feelings, problems of scientific objectivity arise. Says behavioral observations sometimes reveal more than verbalizations, and that better care for the dying can result from studies.

163. ______ . "Problems in the Care of the Dying." *Journal of Chronic Diseases*, 17, no. 2:201-205, 1971.

Says those concerned with evaluation in this area may be biased by their own emotions. Notes published articles giving advice on remembered experiences outnumber those attempting to measure treatment success or failure; need for more research. Cited research reports include own study cited in Entry A-160.

164. _____ . "Talking with People About to Die." *British Medical Journal,* 3:25-27, July 6, 1974.
Reports on interviews with 60 patients dying of cancer who expressed opinions about ways staff spoke to them of their illness. Sees as pertinent the finding that 12 of the 60 "approved the policy of reticence and denial about their fatal illness."

165. HISCOE, Susan. "The Awesome Decision." *American Journal of Nursing*, 73:291-293, February, 1973. Also in *Dying and Grief: Nursing Interventions*, pp. 88-92 (B-45).
Intensive care unit nurse tells of cardiac arrest of 40-year-old man followed by mechanical life maintenance; involvement with wife and family in helping them with decision to stop respirator.

166. HOFFMAN, Esther. "Don't Give Up on Me!" *American Journal of Nursing*, 71:60-62, January, 1971. Also in *The Dying Patient: A Nursing Perspective*, pp. 44-48 (B-6).
Staff nurse relates experiences, shares feeling about three-month period she cared for dying man and worked closely with his wife. Tells how hearing Kubler-Ross two weeks before patient died helped her understand patient's responses.

167. HOFFMAN, James W. "When a Loved One Is Dying. . .How to Decide What to Tell Him." *Today's Health*, 50:40-43, February, 1972.
Presents arguments for and against telling patient of his fatal condition. Comments on Kubler-Ross's work that advocates letting patient do the telling, relating this to personal experience when father and friend were dying.

168. HOLMES, Marguerite J. "Nursing Intervention with a Dying Patient," in *Current Concepts in Clinical Nursing*, Volume 3, edited by Margery Duffey and others. St. Louis: The C.V. Mosby Company, 1971. Pp. 37-47.
Describes situation created by dying woman who evoked strong negative feelings in hospital nursing staff; ways nurse consultant worked with staff and patient to promote positive attitudes and facilitate person-centered care.

169. HOPKINS, Clark. "The Right to Die with Dignity," in *The Dying Patient: A Supportive Approach*, pp. 73-94 (B-8).
Retired professor tells of personal involvement with and sup-

port of proposals that would allow persons to determine their own destiny and prevent life-prolonging measures from being initiated against their will when they wish to die. Comments on obstacles erected by medical profession, the law, and religion.

170. HUMAN, Mildred E. "Death of a Neighbor." *American Journal of Nursing*, 73:1914-1916, November, 1973. Also in *Dying and Grief: Nursing Interventions*, pp. 118-121 (B-45).

In response to request for help, nurse goes to home of slightly known neighbor woman's home and finds neighbor's husband dead. Describes involvement in unexpected death situation and ways she was able to be therapeutic.

171. HUTSCHNECKER, Arnold A. "Personality Factors in Dying Patients," in *The Meaning of Death*, pp. 237-250 (B-19).

Discusses differences in characteristics and personality among patients with cancer and those with cardiac disease; uses clinical examples to show they are going to die, are ready, and retain their basic personality.

172. IMARA, Mwalimu. "Dying as the Last Stage of Growth," in *Death: The Final Stage of Growth*, pp. 147-163 (B-37).

Student chaplain working with Kubler-Ross and dying hospitalized patients illustrates growth concept through report of work with 68-year-old dying woman patient who taught him "what growth during the final stage of life really was." Describes the changes that occurred in this person during the last months of her life that enabled her to reach the stage of acceptance.

173. INGLES, Thelma. "St. Christopher's Hospice." *Nursing Outlook*, 22:759-763, December, 1974. Also in *Dying and Grief: Nursing Interventions*, pp. 34-41 (B-45).

Nurse consultant serving as voluntary staff nurse for three weeks discovers how dying patients and their families can be helped. Comments on physical, emotional care; paired nursing; ways staff support each other, families, patients; activities upon patient death; outpatient services; role of volunteers.

174. JACKSON, Nancy A. "A Child's Preoccupation with Death," in *ANA Clinical Sessions: American Nurses' Association, 1968 Dallas*. New York: Appleton-Century-Crofts, 1968. Pp. 172-179.

Nurse notes literature regarding children's death concepts,

describes their manifestations in eight-year-old with poor prognosis to whom she gave intensive nursing care two hours daily for a month. Summarizes from experience implications for nurses working with hospitalized children.

175. JACKSON, Pat L. "The Child's Developing Concept of Death: Implications for Nursing Care of the Terminally Ill." *Nursing Forum*, 14, no. 2:204-215, 1975.

Outlines development stages from infancy through adolescence and discusses the evolving and accompanying death concepts nurses need to know about for providing dying children and adolescents with effective nursing care. Cites 14 references.

176. JANZEN, Erica. "Relief of Pain: Prerequisite to the Care and Comfort of the Dying." *Nursing Forum*, 13, no. 1:48-51, 1974.

Comments on way this chief cause of suffering is diminished or relieved through individualized analgesic regimen, which may include heroin, gin, or cocaine, at St. Christopher's Hospice, London.

177. JOHNSON, Joan Marie. "Stillbirth – A Personal Experience." *American Journal of Nursing*, 72:1595-1596, September, 1972.

Nurse-patient describes impact of staff's unconcern. Uses Engel's stages of grief to describe personal responses suggesting helping actions nurses can offer mothers who have lost their child.

178. JOSEPH, Florence. "Transference and Countertransference in the Case of a Dying Patient." *Psychoanalysis and the Psychoanalytic Review*, 49, no. 4:21-34, 1962.

Psychoanalyst reports personal struggles with feelings about involvement in conspiracy with patient's significant others to shield her from knowledge of impending death from cancer. Raises questions about proper professional actions, interprets behavior, describes verbal/nonverbal communication between self and patient.

179. KALISH, Richard A. "The Onset of the Dying Process." *Omega*, 1:57-69, February, 1970.

Considers ways people learn of their dying condition; suggests three catagories of informational input that lead to awareness. Identifies and discusses eight tasks of dying persons and indicates professionals' role in assisting patients to accomplish them.

180. KARON, Myron and Joel Vernick. "An Approach to Emotional Support of Fatally Ill Children." *Clinical Pediatrics*, 7: 274-280, May, 1968.

Describes National Cancer Institute research involving 51 patients between 9 and 20 with acute leukemia; use of "life space" interviews, weekly group sessions; information meetings with pediatrician; parents' meetings to facilitate communication among patients, parents, care providers.

181. KASPER, August M. "The Doctor and Death," in *The Meaning of Death*, pp. 259-270 (B-19).

Discusses physicians' attitudes toward death and the dying; consequences of training that stresses "scientific objectivity"; ways surgeons and psychiatrists protect themselves; physicians' reluctance to make or reveal serious diagnoses.

182. KASTENBAUM, Robert. "The Child's Understanding of Death: How Does it Develop? in *Explaining Death to Children,* pp. 89-108 (B-27).

Notes imprecision though usefulness of guidelines for mental, emotional, social growth. Comments on close relationship of general intellectual development to ideas regarding death. Discusses behaviors and experiences that accompany evolution of understanding from infancy through adolescence.

183. KAZZAZ, David S. and Raymond Vickers. "Geriatric Staff Attitudes Toward Death." *Journal of American Geriatrics Society*, 16:1364-1371, December, 1968. Also in *Confrontations of Death*, pp. 98-103 (B-54).

Reports findings of study done to determine how feelings about and reactions to dying and death affected patient care. Discusses educational approaches used; how psychodrama demonstrated contrast between staff, patient attitudes; how staff's ability to understand own feelings and talk openly with patients occurred.

184. KLAGSBRUN, Samuel C. "Cancer, Nurses, and Emotions." *RN Magazine*, 33:46-51, January, 1970.

Content, except for deletion of several paragraphs and colleague's commentary, same as "Cancer, Emotions, and Nurses" cited in Entry A-185.

185. ______ . "Cancer, Emotions, and Nurses." *American Journal of Psychiatry*, 126:71-78, March, 1970. Also in *The Psy-*

chodynamics of Patient Care, by Lawrence H. Schwartz and Jane L. Schwartz. Englewood Cliffs, N. J.: Prentice-Hall, 1972. Pp. 294-304.

Psychiatrist describes small cancer research unit and efforts to improve patient care and management; how weekly meetings with nurses helped them share concerns, feelings, anxieties, and see patients as people; self-care experiment nurses initiated and its effect on patients and staff. Commentary by John Reckless follows.

186. ______ . "Communications in the the Treatment of Cancer." *American Journal of Nursing*, 71:944-948, May, 1971. Also in *Nursing and the Cancer Patient*, pp. 84-91 (B-7). Available from American Cancer Society.

Discusses obstacles cancer patients needing to understand their illness meet when trying to find out what is wrong; factors contributing to huge vacuum in emotional care. Illustrates need for open communication with clinical examples.

187. KLERMAN, Gerald L. "Drugs and the Dying Patient," in *Psychopharmacologic Agents for the Terminally Ill and Bereaved*, pp. 14-27 (B-26).

Reviews use of psychopharmacologic drugs as research and therapeutic tools for dying patients in: relieving and lessening pain; potentiating narcotics and analgesics; reducing anxiety and depression; psychedelic approaches to help patients encounter death. Discusses implications of drug use. Cites 44 references.

188. KLIMAN, Gilbert. "The Child Faces His Own Death," in *Death and Bereavement*, edited by Austin H. Kutscher. Springfield, Ill.: Charles C Thomas, Publisher, 1969. Pp 20-27.

Comments on hazards inherent in shielding children from reality of death. Describes disruptive emotional symptoms in four-year-old boy following leukemia diagnosis. Relates how pet's death provided opportunity for mother and son to talk openly of death, which fostered development of truthful talk with one another

189. KLOPF, Joan K. "Please Don't Go Away: A Crisis When Nobody Intervened." *Nursing Clinics of North America*, 9:77-80, March, 1974.

Nurse-patient has baby that dies at birth. Describes her grief, distress, and the avoidance behavior of nursing staff, who ignored her emotional needs.

190. KNEISL, Carol Ren. "Dying Patients and Their Families: How Staff Can Give Support." *Hospital Topics*, 45:37-39, November, 1967.

Identifies factors contributing to dying patients' loneliness, abondonment, isolation. Suggests measures for enhancing care: including patient/family in care planning; providing consistent, limited numbers of care-giving personnel; tailoring visiting privileges; facilitating anticipatory grieving; assisting staff and family to cope with emotions and crisis of death.

191. ______ . "Thoughtful Care for the Dying." *American Journal of Nursing,* 68:550-553, March, 1968. Also in *The Dying Patient: A Nursing Perspective*, pp. 148-156 (B-6).

Discusses death-related taboos in hospitals; how hospitals' policies and practices contribute to patients' loneliness, isolation, feelings of abandonment; defenses nurses use to protect selves from involvement; serious obstacles in providing care created by inadequate communication among health team members. Suggests actions for providing more effective care.

192. ______ . "Grieving: A Response to Loss," in *The Dying Patient: A Supportive Approach*, pp. 31-46 (B-8).

Discussion on grieving process refers to Lindemann and Engel; considers anticipatory grieving and describes behaviors and situations nurses must be aware of for effective intervention in work with families before and/or after loss of a loved one through death.

193. KNOX, Merrily F. ". . .And the Cells Grow." *American Journal of Nursing*, 70:1047, May, 1970. Also in *Nursing and the Cancer Patient*, pp. 113-114 (B-7).

Initially shocked at conspiracy of silence surrounding 20-year-old cancer patient, nurse later believes patient had right *not* to know.

194. KNUDSON, Alfred G. and Joseph M. Natterson. "Participation of Parents in the Hospital Care of Fatally Ill Children." *Pediatrics*, 26:482-491, September, 1960.

Describes facilities, philosophy, development of parent participation program at City of Hope Medical Center. Comments on benefits for patients, parents, staff; how children under six benefited most; how participating in child's care helped parents cope with own anxieties, feelings.

195. KNUTSON, Andie L. "Cultural Beliefs on Life and Death," in *The Dying Patient*, pp. 42-64 (B-5).

Notes multiple conceptual themes about meaning of death; importance of definitions; how death is depersonalized. Comments on ways individual worth is evaluated by health and medical professionals; how this influences life-death decisions. Discusses effects of societal changes on peoples' experiences with and attitudes about dying, death. Touches on communication with patients about death.

196. KOBRZYCKI, Paula. "Dying with Dignity at Home." *American Journal of Nursing*, 75:1312-1313, August, 1975. Also in *Dying and Grief; Nursing Interventions*, pp. 17-21 (B-45).

Description of hospital staff's involvement in teaching family of 22-year-old Vietnam veteran about care techniques and prescribed treatments so he could be taken home to die in their care.

197. KOENIG, Ronald R. "Dying vs. Well-Being." *Omega*, 4, no. 3:181-194, 1973. Also in *Nursing Digest*, 2:49-54, May, 1974. Also in *Nursing Digest: 1975 Focus on Care of the Elderly*, pp. 108-113; *Nursing Digest: 1975 Review of Medicine and Surgery*, pp. 147-152; *Nursing Digest: 1975 Review of Psychiatry and Mental Health*, pp. 115-160. Wakefield, Mass.: Contemporary Publishing, 1975.

Believes the quality of life, not its length is pertinent, and patient's own criteria must determine what is important to him. Says physical pain, emotional pain, isolation, loneliness can be more threatening than death. Notes importance of touch; how death's uncertainty can be reassuring. Offers suggestions for communicating with patients about dying.

198. KOOP, C. Everett. "The Seriously Ill or Dying Child: Supporting the Patient and the Family." *Pediatric Clinics of North America*, 16, no. 3:555-564, 1969.

Surgeon comments on neonatal emergencies, children facing impending death through accidents, acutely ill surgical patients. Focuses on care of chronically ill child when death is inevitable. Offers suggestions for answering parents' questions. Discusses palliative measures for dying child, getting autopsy permission.

199. KOVACS, Liberty. "A Personal Perspective of Death and Dying," in *The Nurse as Caregiver for the Terminal Patient and His Family*, pp. 160-167 (B-12).

Nurse blocks suicide attempt of long-term patient early in her career and tells of subsequent efforts to prepare self to confront the realities of dying and death in developing a perspective of death that has place in her life as a person and a nurse.

200. KRANT, Melvin J. "The Organized Care of the Dying Patient." *Hospital Practice*, 7:101-108, January, 1972.

Describes oncological unit designed to support patients' need to "die well" through in-hospital, outpatient, home care services. Care philosophy illustrated by clinical example. Discusses: problems involved in telling patient of condition; allowing patient to react to his perceived reality; staff's interpersonal involvement with patients.

201. ______ . "In the Context of Dying," in *Psychosocial Aspects of Terminal Care,* pp. 201-209 (B-52).

Discusses problems, issues in care of dying persons. Considers cost power in medical spheres; deficiencies in medical, nursing, social work education; sex-limited professional rules; physicians' defensive depersonalization; hospitals' focus on acutely ill.

202. KRANT, Melvin J. and Alan Sheldon. "The Dying Patient – Medicine's Responsibility." *Journal of Thanatology*, 1:1-24, January/February, 1971.

Considers multiplicity of problems involved in dying patients' care. Discusses dying process in modern hospitals. Notes interaction between patient, family, physician, and staff; impact of death upon families. Describes family therapy unit as integral part of oncology service. Offers suggestions for care of the dying and those surrounding, surviving them. Cites 59 references.

203. KRON, Joan. "Designing a Better Place to Die." *New York Magazine*, 9:43-49, March 1, 1976.

Presents architect's sketches with description of and rationale for physical environment of Connecticut Hospice, which incorporates philosophy and care concepts of St. Christopher's Hospice with those of nurse Florence Wald and other health care professionals.

204. KUBLER-ROSS, Elisabeth. "Coping Patterns of Patients Who Know Their Diagnosis," in *Catastrophic Illness in the Seventies: Critical Issues and Complex Decisions.* Proceedings of the Fourth National Symposium. New York: The National Cancer Foundation, 1970. Pp. 14-19.

Comments on our death-denying society; says patients know when they are dying and can teach others. Discusses, gives examples of five stages of dying. Notes how denial, anger, and acceptance affect family. Differentiates kinds of hope.

205. ______ . "The Dying Patient's Point of View," in *The Dying Patient*, pp. 156-170 (B-5).

Brief history of author's work with dying patients. Uses two specific situations to illustrate patients' need to share feelings about their fatal diagnoses. Emphasizes importance of listening to patients and of accepting them as they are. Discusses common denominators of shock and disbelief, anger, bargaining, depression, acceptance.

206. ______ . "What Is It Like to Be Dying?" *American Journal of Nursing,* 71: 54-61, January, 1971. Also in *The Dying Patient: A Nursing Perspective*, pp. 33-43 (B-6).

Comments on our death-denying society; contrasts dying at home in former years with dying in hospitals today. Tells what can be learned from dying patients; illustrates importance of *now*. Describes and gives examples of denial, anger, bargaining, depression, and acceptance, noting stages not necessarily sequential.

207. ______ . "Dying with Dignity." *The Canadian Nurse*, 67:31-35, October, 1971.

Author tells how her interest in dying patients began; of first patient from whom she learned importance of *now*. Notes three kinds of language patients use in talk about dying; need to provide patient with hope. Provides clinical examples to illustrate stages of dying. Considers issue of life prolongation.

208. ______ . "Anger Before Death." *Nursing 71*, 1: 12-14, December, 1971.

Says dying situation especially difficult for family and hospital staff when patient displaces and projects anger. Suggests means nurses can use in coping with patient's anger, using clinical examples to illustrate influence of nurse responses on patient behavior.

209. ______ . "Facing up to Death." *Today's Education*, 61: 30-32, January, 1972.

Briefly discusses stages of dying; how patients helped students face their own death fears. Tells of need for death education; ways to assist children face reality of own death, help siblings of dying patients.

210. ______. "The Right to Die with Dignity." *Bulletin of the Menninger Clinic*, 36: 302-312, May, 1972.

General comments on depersonalized, mechanized care of dying patients in hospitals. Tells how work with dying began; that interviews with 500 patients indicate importance of providing hope and assurance of not being deserted. Briefly outlines five stages of dying. Uses clinical examples to exemplify dying with dignity.

211. ______. "Hope and the Dying Patient." *Psychosocial Aspects of Terminal Care*, pp. 221-226 (B-52).

Comments on games people play when faced with dying person and on patient's need for "hope and reassurance that he will not be deserted." Describes how hope of the dying differs from that of healthy people.

212. ______. "On the Use of Psychopharmacologic Agents for the Dying Patient and the Bereaved," in *Psychopharmacologic Agents for the Terminally Ill and Bereaved*, pp. 3-6 (B-26).

Acknowledges usefulness of these agents but suggests that too often they are used to accommodate the professional's own needs or discomforts, to sedate an angry patient or relative, or to avoid interpersonal involvement.

213. ______. "The Languages of the Dying Patients." *Humanitas*, 10: 5-8, February, 1974.

Notes "plain English" and verbal and nonverbal symbolical languages are used. Story of eight-year-old girl in oxygen tent illustrates symbolical verbal language; kidney transplant candidate of 13 who "shot" girls with healthy kidneys depicts use of symbolical nonverbal language.

214. ______. "Death as Part of My Own Personal Life," in *Death: The Final Stage of Growth*, pp. 119-126 (B-37).

Shares life experiences which contributed to "making me what I am" and may have led author to field of dying and death, molded her views on death and life.

215. KUHN, Margaret E. "Death and Dying: The Right to Live – The Right to Die," in *ANA Clinical Sessions: American Nurses' Association, 1974 San Francisco*. New York: Appleton-Century-Crofts, 1975. Pp. 184-189.

Retired nurse's observations about attitudes toward death and impact of medical technology on keeping people alive. Identifies ten issues concerning dying and death. Views nurses as advocates of aged and dying. Asks for assistance in bringing about change.

216. KURTAGH, Cathryn. "Willie's Drunk and Nellie's Dying; There Ain't Nobody Free." *Nursing Forum*, 11, no. 2: 221-224, 1972.

Relates personal experiences in situations involving dying and death; says nurses must "include the family in whatever ways they can . . . to contribute to the dying patient's well-being" and collaborate with other health professionals in helping families cope.

217. KUTSCHER, Austin H. "The Psychosocial Aspects of the Oral Care of the Dying Patient," in *Psychosocial Aspects of Terminal Care,* pp. 126-141 (B-52).

Discusses importance of mouth care, considering pain, psychogenic components, drooling, odor, medication side effects, psychological problems of oral disturbances and their impact upon patient.

218. LACASSE, Christine M. "A Dying Adolescent." *American Journal of Nursing,* 75:433-434, March, 1975. Also in *Contemporary Nursing Series: Nursing of Children and Adolescents,*compiled by Andrea B. O'Connor. New York: American Journal of Nursing Company, 1975. Pp. 249-253.

Comments on ways age/stage of emotional growth and development affect how 16-year-old boy deals with acute leukemia.

219. LASAGNA, Louis. "A Person's Right to Die." *Johns Hopkins Magazine*, 59, no. 2: 34-41, 1968. Also in *Confrontations of Death*, pp. 109-110 (B-54).

Says whether to prolong existence of terminal patients mechanically is most difficult problem facing physicians. Comments on ordinary versus extraordinary life-preserving measures, euthanasia.

220. ______ . "Physicians' Behavior Toward the Dying Patient," in *The Dying Patient*, pp. 83-101 (B-5).

Contends physicians are influenced by patient's age, social worth, ability to pay, attractiveness, and by appeal of disease, physician's own optimism or pessimism, orientation toward conservative or radical approaches. Discusses factors influencing prognosis, patient care; euthanasia. Includes letter on patients' right to die.

221. ______ . "The Prognosis of Death," in *The Dying Patient*, pp. 67-82 (B-5).

Defines terminal illness. Discusses factors influencing prognostic accuracy, including medical competency, available therapeutic modalities, time variables, stage of illness. Comments on: variety of physician responses to treatment approaches; informing patient, family; patients' reactions to knowledge of diagnosis.

222. LeSHAN, Lawrence. "Psychotherapy and the Dying Patient," in *Death and Dying*, pp. 28-48 (B-47).

Holds that therapy needs to focus on increasing patient's will to live and on assisting patient to become concerned with his own inner development. Emphasizes importance of *now*; need for therapist to listen carefully, accept what patient says, examine own goals and values, focus upon patient's strengths.

223. ______ . "Mobilizing the Life Force." *Annals of the New York Academy of Sciences*, 164: 847-861, December 19, 1969.

Content essentially same as "Psychotherapy and the Dying Patient" cited in Entry A-222, with audience discussion following paper's presentation added.

224. LeSHAN, Lawrence and Eda LeShan. "Psychotherapy and the Patient with a Limited Life Span." *Psychiatry*, 24: 318-324, November, 1961. Also in *The Interpretation of Death*, pp. 106-115 (B-50).

Explains how psychotherapy with dying patient differs from conventional therapy. Discusses emphasis upon here and now. Focus is upon life, not death, in patient's search for self.

225. LEVINE, Sol and Norman A. Scotch. "Dying as an Emerging Social Problem," in *The Dying Patient*, pp. 211-224 (B-5).

Explains dying and death as problems of different orders with different social impacts. Focuses on management of dying process considering rights of patients, stresses of their families, difficulties they pose for hospitals. Discusses how new medical technologies increase possibility of extending lives but also increase dilemmas.

226. LEWIS, Eloise R. and Esther K. Sump. "Sympathy and Objectivity in Balance," in *Should the Patient Know the Truth*? pp. 115-119 (B-58).

Says question must be individualized by considering attitudes of patient, nurse, physician. Emphasizes need for listening, knowing what information patient possesses, increasing communication between nurses and physicians.

227. LEWIS, Wilma R. "A Time to Die." *Nursing Forum*, 4, no. 1: 6-27, 1965. Also in *The Psychodynamics of Patient Care*, by Lawrence H. Schwartz and Jane L. Schwartz. Englewood Cliffs, N.J.: Prentice-Hall, 1972. Pp. 388-399.

Describes small study aimed at identifying nursing care factors that help lessen physical/emotional distress in dying patients. Presents two patient care situations. Suggests ways to enhance care.

228. LINDEMANN, Erich. "Symptomatology and Management of Acute Grief." *American Journal of Psychiatry*, 101: 141-148, September, 1944. Also in *Death and Identity*, pp. 186-201 (B-20). Also in *Crisis Intervention: Selected Readings*, edited by Howard J. Parad. New York: Family Service Association of America, 1965. Pp. 7-21. Also in *Grief: Selected Readings*. Journal Reprint Series, edited and compiled by Arthur C. Carr and others. New York: Health Sciences Publishing Corporation, 1975. Pp. 85-92. Also in *Death and Identity*, revised edition, pp. 210-221 (B-21).

Classic study on the process of grief based on observations of 101 patients. Describes symptomatology and course of normal grief reactions and morbid grief reactions. Discusses importance of proper management of grief syndrome.

229. LIPPINCOTT, Richard C. "The Physician's Responsibility to the Dying Patient." *Medical Clinics of North America*, 56: 677-680, May, 1970.

Notes attitudes related to appropriateness of a person's death; cites conflicts in patient, physician, health team, and family relationships; lists what caring for dying patients requires of physician.

230. LOWENBERG, June S. "The Coping Behaviors of Fatally Ill Adolescents and Their Parents." *Nursing Forum*, 9, no. 3: 269-287, 1970.

Remarks on coping behaviors in general; focuses on characteristics of approach and avoidance (denial) behavior. Includes lists of behavior indices as "a beginning assessment tool," explaining how used to determine where parents of 13-year-old were in grieving process. Describes situation involving dying 16-year-old and his parents to illustrate coping behaviors.

231. ______ . "Working Through Feelings Around Death," in *The Nurse as Caregiver for the Terminal Patient and His Family*, pp. 125-139 (B-12).

Focuses on need for nurses to examine, acknowledge, and begin to come to terms with their own feelings about dying and death in order to recognize and respond to needs of dying patients.

232. LOWREY, John J. "Changing Concepts of Death." *AORN Journal*, 15: 91-96, February, 1972.

Discusses medical advances that give physicians ability to alter and maintain life. Comments on moral, ethical, legal issues involved in changing death concepts; proposed death definitions; dying patient's "qualified right to refuse treatment."

233. McCUSKER, Sister M. "Gracias, Dinora." *American Journal of Nursing*, 72: 250-252, February, 1972.

English-speaking nurse describes relationship with dying Spanish-speaking, straightforward, five-year-old child. Tells of trust established; ways they communicated with minimum use of words; personal grief at child's death.

234. McDONALD, Molly. "Farewell to a Friend." *American Journal of Nursing*, 68: 733, April, 1968. Also in *The Dying Patient: A Nursing Perspective*, pp. 268-269 (B-6).

Vignette of aging ill man taken from his home and loving wife's care to depersonalized hospital situation where he died alone.

235. McLENAHAN, Irene G. "Helping the Mother Who Has No Baby to Take Home." *American Journal of Nursing*, 62: 70-71, April, 1962.

Describes emotional impact of infant's stillbirth or neonatal death on mothers, and difficulties nurses experience in caring for them.

236. McNULTY, Barbara J. "St. Christopher's Outpatients." *American Journal of Nursing*, 71: 2328-2330, December, 1971. Also in *The Dying Patient: A Nursing Perspective*, pp. 257-263 (B-6).

Describes supportive, advisory home care program that is link between Hospice admission, discharge, readmission, and has liaison with community facilities that provide actual nursing care services for patients while at home.

237. ______ . "Continuity of Care." *British Medical Journal*, 1: 38-39, January 6, 1973.

Reports on work with and services provided to St. Christopher's outpatients during three-year period of research and development project involving 784 patients.

238. MADDISON, David and Beverley Raphael. "The Family of the Dying Patient," in *Psychosocial Aspects of Terminal Care*, pp. 185-200 (B-52).

Comments on complex dynamics involved in work with dying patients' families. Discusses reactions of individual family members and of the family group; implications current knowledge has for health care practice and intervention. Cites 31 references.

239. MAGUIRE, Daniel C. "The Freedom to Die." *Commonweal*, 96: 423-427, August 11, 1972.

Questions when terminating life of dying person by active means or benign neglect is a moral procedure; focuses on irreversibly comatose patient and right of conscious patient with artificially supported life to stop treatment.

240. ______ . "Death by Chance, Death by Choice." *Atlantic Monthly*, 221: 57-65, January, 1974. Also in *Nursing Digest*, 2: 36-42, October, 1974. Also in *Nursing Digest: 1975 Focus on Care of the Elderly*, pp. 48-54; *Nursing Digest: 1975 Review of Medicine and Surgery*, pp. 175-181. Wakefield, Mass.: Contemporary Publishing, 1975.

Theologian discusses how advances in science and medical technology have complicated definition of death. Raises moral, ethical, legal questions regarding acts of commission or omission in prolonging life or hastening death.

241. MALITZ, Sidney and Eda G. Goldstein. "Psychotherapy and Pharmacotherapy in a Dying Patient: Report of a Supervised Case," in *Psychopharmacologic Agents for the Terminally Ill and Bereaved*, pp. 189-201 (B-26).

Nine-page report identical to the one presented by Goldstein and Malitz cited in Entry A-128. Discussion of report enlarged.

242. MANGEN, Sister Francis. "Psychological Aspects of Nursing the Advanced Cancer Patient." *Nursing Clinics of North America*, 2: 649-658, December, 1967.

Describes atmosphere of hope at Calvary Hospital where nursing goal is comfort, not recovery. Discusses measures used to alleviate anxiety, control pain; importance of touch, listening, respecting denial, providing opportunity for expressing feelings.

242a MANT, A. Keith. "The Medical Definition of Death," in *Man's Concern with Death,* pp. 13-24 (B-63). Also in *Death: Current Perspectives,* pp. 218-231 (B-56).

Discusses the diagnosis of death, modern criteria of death, and importance of determining exact moment of death in relation to organ transplantation and artificial prolongation of life.

243. MARKS, Mary J. "The Grieving Patient and His Family." *American Journal of Nursing*, 76: 1488-1491, September, 1976. Also in *Dying and Grief: Nursing Interventions*, pp. 95-99 (B-45).

Commentary on grieving presents factors to consider for helpful nurse action. Treatment of topic superficial.

244. MARTINSON, Beatrice. "Must It Be?" *American Journal of Nursing*, 71:1887, September, 1970.

Hospital rules and rigid nurse behavior prevent woman from being with 80-year-old dying mother.

245. MARTINSON, Ida M. "Why Don't We Let Them Die at Home?" *RN Magazine*, 39: 58-65, January, 1976.

Nurse reports work with parents of eight children who died at home. Describes nursing interventions with one of these dying children and reports benefits to child and to family.

246. MASCO, Sister Josephine. "This One Was Different." *American Journal of Nursing,* 67:1898-1902, September, 1967.

Senior nursing student describes unexpected stillborn delivery of a mother she followed through pregnancy, labor, delivery, and postpartum care. Tells about the nursing interventions used to help the woman and her husband deal with the tragedy.

247. MAUKSCH, Hans O. "The Organizational Context of Dying," in *Death: The Final Stage of Growth*, pp. 7-24 (B-37).

Characterizes hospitals as efficient impersonal institutions committed to the healing process, not to human needs of sick people. Discusses why hospitals rarely are responsive to special needs of dying patients and explores the reasons for the constraints existing in hospitals today.

248. MAXWELL, Sister Marie. "A Terminally Ill Adolescent and Her Family and How Staff Members Helped Them and Each Other." *American Journal of Nursing*, 72:925-927, May, 1972. Also in *The Dying Patient: A Nursing Perspective*, pp. 233-237 (B-6).

Nurse describes initial efforts to respect parents' wish not to inform their 16-year-old daughter of her prognosis despite cues from patient indicating her desire to know truth. Discusses how staff and parents were prepared for dealing with an aware adolescent on her readmission to hospital and how communication was facilitated.

249. MEAD, Margaret. "The Right to Die." *Nursing Outlook*, 16: 20-21, October, 1968. Also in *The Dying Patient: A Nursing Perspective*, pp. 12-14 (B-6).

Anthropologist notes how new medical knowledge and skills complicate dying process and bring fear of being "kept alive" without being humanly related. Believes nurses/physicians must remain pledged to sustain life; suggests ways individuals can express their right not to be saved.

250. MEINHART, Noreen T. "The Cancer Patient: Living in the Here and Now." *Nursing Outlook,* 16:64-69, May, 1968. Also in *Nursing and the Cancer Patient,* pp. 61-74 (B-7).

Discusses significance of attitudes toward symptoms and ways attitudes are influenced by diagnosis, treatment, prognosis, personal relationships, religion, race, socioeconomic status, education.

251. MERVYN, Frances. "The Plight of Dying Patients in Hospitals." *American Journal of Nursing*, 71: 1988-1990, October, 1971. Also in *The Dying Patient: A Nursing Perspective*, pp. 63-69 (B-6).

Comments on care of dying in general hospitals where patient often must fend for himself and has little meaningful communication with staff. Identifies factors that influence patient care.

252. MEYER, Bernard C. "Should the Patient Know the Truth?" *Journal of the Mount Sinai Hospital*, 20: 344-350, March/April, 1954.

Explores complex nature of truth telling with examples of positive and negative consequences. Says cancer diagnosis presents greatest problem. Opposes establishment of truth-telling policies.

253. ______ . "What Patient, What Truth?" in *Should the Patient Know the Truth*? pp. 47-58 (B-58).

Reprint of "Should the Patient Know the Truth?" cited in Entry A-252.

254. MILES, Margaret S. "Carl and Willy." *Nursing Forum*, 8, no. 2:146-150, 1969.

Vignette regarding staff feelings and reactions to dying and death of teenaged boy named Carl; how in failing to tell fellow patient Willy of his death, they "in a way . . . lost Willy too."

255. MILLER, Michael B. "Decision-Making in the Death Process of the Ill Aged." *Geriatrics*, 26: 105-116, May, 1971.

Describes ten patient-care situations representing common experiences in daily operation of long-term care facility; focuses on decision-making processes involved in preparations for patient's death. Indicates how patient, family, physician, nursing staff, and institution are involved in and affected by decisions.

256. MILLER, Peter G. and Jan Ozga. "How to Answer the Question 'Mommy, What Happens When I Die?' " *Mental Hygiene,* 57:21-22, Spring, 1973. Also in *Nursing Digest,* 2:76-79, May, 1974.

Outlines children's developing concept of death. Lists things *not* to tell a child.

257. MORISON, Robert S. "Dying." *Scientific American*, 229: 54-62, September, 1973.

Discusses ways in which industrialization, advances in science, and medical technology have influenced mortality rates and the places where people die. Comments on: St. Christopher's Hospice; differences between prolonging life and prolonging dying; criteria for definition of death; active/passive euthanasia. Includes sample living will.

258. MORRISSEY, James R. "Death Anxiety in Children with Fatal Illness." *American Journal of Psychotherapy*, 4: 606-615, October, 1964. Also reprinted, with additional formula-

tions, in *Crisis Intervention: Selected Readings*, edited by Howard J. Parad. New York: The Family Service Association of America, 1965. Pp. 324-338.

Reports study of 50 children, admitted to City of Hope Medical Center with leukemia and cancer, to determine age when children experience death anxiety; how expressed and handled; implications of the findings for care of children aware of impending death. Study indicated death anxiety usually seen in children ten or older.

259. MORSE, Joan. "The Goal of Life Enhancement for a Fatally Ill Child." *Children*, 17: 63-68, March/April, 1970.

Describes interdisciplinary teamwork in care of child whose illness involved repeated hospitalizations and follow-up care from age 10 till death at 13.

260. NAGY, Maria H. "The Child's View of Death." *Journal of Genetic Psychology*, 3, no. 1: 3-27, 1948. Also in *The Meaning of Death*, pp. 79-97 (B-19).

Classic, multicited study based on data from 378 Budapest children who wrote compositions or made drawings about death, then discussed them. Findings of three major developmental stages indicate: no definitive idea of death in children under five; between five and nine, death is personified; recognition of death as cessation and inevitable by ninth or tenth year. Presents children's responses.

261. NAKUSHIAN, Janet M. "Restoring Parents' Equilibrium after Sudden Infant Death." *American Journal of Nursing*, 76: 1600-1603, October, 1976.

Describes parental reactions to tragedy; how uninformed physician and nurses compound suffering and guilt; value of public health nurses' informational visits to grieving parents. "Survey: SIDS Research and Counseling" accompanies article.

262. NATTERSON, Joseph M. and Alfred G. Knudson. "Observations Concerning Fear of Death in Fatally Ill Children and Their Mothers." *Psychosomatic Medicine*, 22:456-463, November/December, 1960. Also in *Death and Identity*, pp. 226-239 (B-20).

Reports study findings and identifies influencing factors in behavior of children at City of Hope Medical Center. Children's fear are age-dependent, with separation fears typical from infancy through five; fear of death evident in children ten or older. Describes triphasic response of mothers when illness lasted more than four months, with maximum distress and denial typical of the initial phase and calm acceptance of their child's impending death characterizing the final phase.

263. NEALE, Robert E. "Between the Nipple and the Everlasting Arms." *Archives of the Foundation of Thanatology*, 3, no. 1: 21-30, 1971. Also in *Union Seminary Quarterly Review*, 27: 81-90, Winter, 1972.

Clergyman relates experience with dying man while volunteer chaplain at St. Christopher's Hospice. Gives impressions of care provided; discusses being present through touching, loving, and feeding.

263a NETSKY, Martin G. "Dying in a System of 'Good Care': Case Report and Analysis." The Pharos of Alpha Omega Alpha, 39:57-61, April, 1976. Available from Euthanasia Educational Council.

Physician raises profound questions about hospital care of dying patients. Says what happened to his dying 80-year-old mother "was a nightmare of depersonalized institutionalization," of rote management presumably related to science, and based on the team approach of subdivision of work.

264. NICHOLS, Elizabeth G. "Jeannette: No Hope for Cure." *Nursing Forum*, 11, no. 1: 97-104, 1972.

Describes nursing care provided dying young mother of two. Discusses difficulty in switching from recovery to comfort care goals, importance of understanding grieving process, what comfort care was involved, and the risk the work involved for nurse.

265. NIELSEN, Sharon. "Home Visiting for Patients Receiving Special Care." *Nursing Clinics of North America*, 7: 383-387, June, 1972.

Describes oncology-hematology unit project where nurses initiated own visits to discharged patients. Comments on beneficial effects of home visits; how hope changes; comfort measures used.

266. NORTHRUP, Fran C. "The Dying Child." *American Journal of Nursing*, 74:1066-1068, June, 1974. Also in *Dying and Grief: Nursing Interventions*, pp. 11-16 (B-45).

Indicates importance of meeting child's basic physical (comfort) needs and emotional (caring) needs in facilitating ultimate goal of communication. Offers suggestions for enhancing care, involving parents and siblings.

267. NORTON, Janice. "Treatment of a Dying Patient," in *The Psychoanalytic Study of the Child*, Volume XVIII, edited by Ruth S. Eissler and others. New York: International Universities Press, 1963. Also in *The Interpretation of Death,* pp. 19-38 (B-50).

Psychiatrist reports intensive work with 32-year-old woman for three months preceding her death. Discusses analytic components, patient's defense mechanisms, disrupted interpersonal relationships. Demonstrates own human involvement, including quiet presence and rendering physical care. Describes patient's regression, depression, problems related to loss, ways of managing anxiety.

268. NOYES, Russel, Jr. "The Care and Management of the Dying." *Archives of Internal Medicine*, 128:299-303, August, 1971.

Outlines traditional concepts of appropriate dying; notes contemporary differences. Discusses: psychological reactions to dying; relieving pain, other symptoms; involving patient, family in treatment decisions; effective communications; providing support.

269. OERLEMANS, Marguerite. "Eli." *American Journal of Nursing*, 72: 1440-1441, August, 1972.

Nurse shares her feelings and reactions to dying/death of 33-year-old man "too young to die" and the need she had for personal support in her grief.

270. OKEN, Donald. "What to Tell Cancer Patients: A Study of Medical Attitudes." *Journal of the American Medical Association,* 175:1120-1128, April 1, 1961.

Frequently cited study involving survey of 219 physicians asked to indicate how and/or what they told cancer patients about their condition; ninety percent preferred telling patient nothing about malignancy. Includes questionnaire used, discussion of findings, comments on prior surveys.

271. OLSEN, Emily. "Effect of Nurse-Patient Interaction on a Terminal Patient." *ANA Clinical Sessions: American Nurses'*

Association, 1968 Dallas. New York: Appleton-Century-Crofts, 1968. Pp. 90-94.

Describes how show of genuine interest and willingness to understand a dying 72-year-old women helped patient talk about distressing feelings and work through grief and face death.

272. ORAFTIK, Nancy. "Only Time to Touch." *Nursing Forum,* 11, no. 2: 205-213, 1972.

Senior nursing student shares experience of providing for emotional needs of depressed 21-year-old man dying of leukemia.

273. ORBACH, Charles E., Arthur M. Sutherland, and Mary F. Bozeman. "The Psychological Impact of Cancer and Its Treatment: III. The Adaptation of Mothers to the Threatened Loss of Their Children Through Leukemia: Part II." *Cancer,* 8: 20-33, January/February, 1955. Available from American Cancer Society. For Part I see Entry A-46.

Reports on analysis of TAT responses of 20 mothers in study; verbatim replies illustrate themes elicited. Theoretical discussion focusing on mother-daughter relationship stems from surprising finding of maternal grandmothers' nonsupport of own daughters who faced a child's impending death. Summary and recommendations for both parts of report; suggests ways nurses can enhance care

274. PACYNA, Dorothy A. "Response to a Dying Child." *Nursing Clinics of North America,* 5:421-430, September, 1970.

Discusses dying five-year-old boy's need for support; deals with his fears of aloneness, intrusive procedures, death. Describes nursing actions; parents' reactions to situation. Applies general systems theory approach to nurse-child-parent relationship.

275. PALEN, Charity S. "The Passage." *American Journal of Nursing,* 75: 2004-2005, November, 1975. Also in *Dying and Grief: Nursing Interventions,* pp. 48-50 (B-45).

Nursing student tells of emotional turmoil and physical revulsion experienced in efforts to resuscitate guest at wedding whose heart arrested.

276. PATTISON, E. Mansell. "The Experience of Dying." *American Journal of Psychotherapy,* 21:32-43, January, 1967.

Comments on complexity of dying and three types of attitudes toward it; how dying experience is conditioned by age and human feelings that transcend culture, society, beliefs. Views death as crisis event characterized by five criteria. Outlines ways to help dying persons. Discusses what constitutes appropriate death.

277. PITKIN, Dorothy. "One Woman's Death – A Victory and a Triumph," in *Death: The Final Stage of Growth*, pp. 105-116 (B-37).

Last writing of once self-sufficient author describes final days in a nursing home. Introduction by son comments on his mother's philosophy and graceful, dignified death at 75.

278. POI, Kathleen M. "Who Cared About Tony?" *American Journal of Nursing*, 72: 1848-1851, October, 1972.

Describes how nursing staff discovered they were not meeting needs of fatally ill 15-year-old or his parents, and steps taken to remedy situation in hospitalization prior to death.

279. PORTER, J. V. "A Therapeutic Community for the Dying." *AORN Journal*, 21:838-839, 842, April 1975.

Clergyman presents variety of ideas related to dying persons. Tells of importance of being present, the triple separation of death, giving self permission to die, suppressed and delayed grief.

280. PRATT, Margaret A. "A Hospitalized Preschool Child Copes with a Fatal Illness." *ANA Clinical Sessions: American Nurses' Association, 1968 Dallas*. New York: Appleton-Century-Crofts, 1968. Pp. 190-198.

Nurse describes relationship and nursing intervention with four-year-old boy during hospitalizations and during daily clinic visits until two days before his death at home. Cites examples of child's coping measures; tells of work with boy's mother.

281. PROULX, John R. "Ministering to the Dying: A Joint Pastoral and Nursing Effort." *Hospital Progress*, 56:62-63, March, 1975.

Comments on counseling/care components in work with the terminally ill and on contributions nurses and chaplains can make to dying patients' care by transcending traditional roles. Says formal and continuing education has role in developing skills.

282. QUINT, Jeanne C. "The Impact of Mastectomy." *American Journal of Nursing*, 63:88-92, November, 1963. Also in *The*

Psychodynamics of Patient Care by Lawrence H. Schwartz and Jane L. Schwartz. Englewood Cliffs, N.J.: Prentice-Hall, 1972. Pp. 256-266. Also in *Nursing and the Cancer Patient,* pp. 340-351 (B-7).

Study on impact of breast surgery on 21 women; problems nurses encountered when providing their care. While not specifically about the dying, fear of and talk about death did arise. Patients' viewpoint gave cues for providing supportive nursing care.

283. ______ . "Institutional Practices of Information Control." *Psychiatry*, 28: 119-132, May, 1965.

Describes research study of action, behavior, and communication tactics of physicians and nurses toward patients with cancer. Interview situation during study permitted patients to talk openly about facing possibility of death alone because family, friends, nurses, and physicians blocked discussion of their fate. Comments on hope rationale used to justify professionals' actions; on cancer as a professional threat; on consequences of information concealment.

284. ______ . "Awareness of Death and the Nurse's Composure." *Nursing Research*, 15, no. 1: 49-55, 1966. Also in *The Dying Patient: A Nursing Perspective*, pp. 164-180 (B-6).

Discusses strategies nurses use to maintain composure when interacting with dying patients. Identifies four kinds of death expectations; defines awareness contexts, "nothing-more-to-do" phase.

285. ______ . "Obstacles to Helping the Dying." *American Journal of Nursing*, 66: 1568-1571, July, 1966. Also in *The Dying Patient: A Nursing Perspective*, pp. 70-77 (B-6).

Considers problems created for hospital nursing staff when patient is not told diagnosis or about dying – patient's behavior does not meet expectations of acceptable dying. Discusses ways dying behaviors and definitions influence attitudes and care practices.

286. ______ . "The Dying Patient: A Difficult Nursing Problem," in *Nursing Clinics of North America*, 7: 736-773, December, 1967.

Considers difficulties associated with work nurses are expected to do and those resulting from personal reactions to the dying process and death in hospital care situations. Suggests ways of lessening the difficulties; ways of dealing with families at death.

287. ______. "When Patients Die: Some Nursing Problems." *Canadian Nurse*, 63: 33-36, December, 1967.

Discusses problems created for nurses when recovery and comfort goals conflict; complications that arise when patients are unaware of their dying situation; factors that contribute to interactional tension between dying patients and nurses; how tension is compounded by paucity of communication between nursing and medical staff. Suggests ways of improving dying patients' care.

288. ______. "The Threat of Death: Some Consequences for Patients and Nurses." *Nursing Forum,* 8, no. 3:286-300, 1969.

Discusses factors relating to depersonalization of dying and death in modern society, their influence on fatally ill persons and on those responsible for their care. Comments on nurse behavior in cardiac and intensive care units where quick decisions about starting life-preserving measure are crux of nurses' work.

289. QUINT, Jeanne C. and Anselm L. Strauss. "Nursing Students, Assignments, and Dying Patients." *Nursing Outlook*, 12: 24-27, January, 1964. Also in *The Dying Patient: A Nursing Perspective*, pp. 187-195 (B-6).

Discusses factors influencing vastly different experiences nurses have with dying patients and death. Describes difficulties students have with dying patients and conditions making their first encounter with dying/death traumatic.

290. RABIN, David L. and Laurel H. Rabin. "Consequences of Death for Physicians, Nurses, and Hospitals," in *The Dying Patient*, pp. 171-208 (B-5).

Notes influence of declining mortality rate on young people's experience with and attitudes toward dying and death. Discusses: how physicians usually cope with dying/death; conflict between physician's roles as member of the social order and of the scientific community. Comments on: hospital staff's effort to send dying patient elsewhere; nurse actions upon death of patient.

291. RAPPAPORT, Sidney C. "Oral Care of the Dying Patient," in *Oral Care of the Aging and Dying Patient*, edited by Austin H. Kutscher and Ivan K. Goldberg. Springfield, Il.: Charles C Thomas, Publisher, 1973. Pp. 92-99. Outlines general and specific needs of the patient based on his disease state and the roles of the dentist, nurse, physician, and family in patient's care.

292. REGAN, Peter F. "The Dying Patient and His Family." *Journal of the American Medical Association*, 192:82-83, May 24, 1965.

Views death as a crisis for patient, family, and physician, and discusses factors that influence successful management of a patient's dying. Suggests ways of diminishing patient's loneliness, apprehension.

293. RICHMOND, Julius B. and Harry A. Weisman. "Psychologic Aspects of Management of Children with Malignant Disease." *American Journal of Diseases of Children,* 89:42-47, January, 1955.

Reports observational study of 48 fatally ill hospitalized children and their parents; indicates child's reaction to illness relates to age of onset. Identifies parents' needs; discusses advantages of parent involvement in child's care and their participation in ward program.

294. RINEAR, Elaine. "The Nurse's Challenge when Death Is Unexpected," *RN Magazine*, 38:50-55, December, 1975.

Nursing care coordinator describes interventions with relatives of persons who were in good health just prior to their unexpected deaths in hospital emergency rooms. Four clinical illustrations.

295. ROBINSON, Lisa. "We Have No Dying Patients." *Nursing Outlook*, 22: 651-653, October, 1974. Also in *Dying and Grief: Nursing Interventions*, pp. 181-188 (B-45).

Nurse teacher describes course designed to help students learn to interact with dying patients; indicates that obstacles and resistance students met from physicians and nurses when they asked to talk with dying patients were similar to those reported by Kubler-Ross (see Entry B-34). Excerpts from students' logs.

296. ROBINSON, Mary E. "When a Child Dies," in *But Not to Lose: A Book of Comfort for Those Bereaved*, edited by Austin H. Kutscher. New York: Fredrick Fell, 1969. Pp. 107-112.

Focuses on reactions and grief experienced by parents and siblings of child who dies after long period of illness. Considers feelings of guilt and ambivalence; anticipatory mourning; children's understanding of death; situational problems arising during course of illness that influence feelings and behaviors of survivors.

297. ROCHLIN, Gregory. "How Younger Children View Death and Themselves," in *Explaining Death to Children*, pp. 51-85 (B-27).

Discusses study that utilized play therapy and conversation with children three to five years of age. Presents four clinical examples to illustrate significant ways children cope with knowledge of death. Includes sample transcrips of conversations with each child.

298. ROOSE, Lawrence J. "To Die Alone." *Mental Hygiene*, 53: 321-326, July, 1969.

Psychiatrist comments on difficulty most physicians have communicating with dying patients; describes family and staff behaviors that isolate patient, adding to his greatest fear – of dying alone. Clinical example illustrates how to facilitate communication.

299. ROSE, Mary A. "Problems Families Face in Home Care." *American Journal of Nursing*, 76: 416-418, March, 1976.

Interviews with families of 26 cancer patients, who were cared for at home until their death, reveals that providing this care created a profound emotional burden for families without nursing assistance.

300. ROSENTHAL, Hattie R. "Psychotherapy for the Dying." *American Journal of Psychotherapy*, 2: 626-633, July 1957. Also in *The Interpretation of Death*, pp. 87-95 (B-50).

Comments on dying person's fears and guilt feelings. Uses vignettes to illustrate how psychotherapy can help to make it easier for the dying to die.

301. SALK, Lee, S.M. Finch and H.S. Belmont. "Sudden Infant Death: Impact on Family and Physician." *Clinical Pediatrics*, 10:248-250, May, 1971. Available from National Foundation for Sudden Infant Death.

Discusses shock of SID for parents and older siblings. Considers the most pervasive emotional reaction "an intense sense of responsible guilt" which presents dilemma for physicians. Comments on benefits of sharing feelings with other parents who experienced similar tragedy.

302. SAUNDERS, Cicely. "The Treatment of Intractable Pain in Terminal Cancer." *Proceedings of the Royal Society of Medicine*, 56: 195-197, March, 1963.

Through analysis of 900 patients' records, identifies cardinal rules for treating pain; advocates giving analgesics "to prevent pain from occurring, not to control it when it is already present." Explains why addiction no problem; emphasizes listening and dealing with patient's mental distress which "may be perhaps the most intractable pain of all."

303. ______ . "The Last Stages of Life." *American Journal of Nursing*, 65: 70-75, March, 1965. Also in *The Dying Patient: A Nursing Perspective*, pp. 247-256 (B-6).

Describes St. Joseph's Hospice, where staff that concentrates on providing symptom relief sees patients as persons in distress. Word portraits illustrate differences in ways patients come to terms with approaching death, ways comfort care is provided. Describes approach to management of pain, chief complaint of patients.

304. ______ . "The Moment of Truth: Care of the Dying Person," in *Death and Dying*, pp. 49-78 (B-47). Also in *Confrontations of Death*, pp. 111-122 (B-54).

Describes work with dying patients in person-centered St. Joseph's Hospice, where success criterion is related to what patient "is *being* in the face of his physical destruction." Discusses: need to recognize difference between treatment and care; prolonging living and prolonging dying; chronic pain and its management; factors to consider when informing patient of condition. Describes ways patient's family is involved; ward dynamics at patient's death.

305. ______ . "The Patient's Response to Treatment. A Photographic Presentation Showing Patients and Their Families," in *Catastrophic Illness in the Seventies: Critical Issues and Complex Decisions.* Proceedings of the Fourth National Symposium. New York: The National Cancer Foundation, 1971. Pp. 33-46.

Words and 35 pictures tell story of care provided dying patients at St. Christopher's Hospice.

306. ______ . "A Therapeutic Community: St. Christophers's Hospice," in *Psychosocial Aspects of Terminal Care,* pp. 275-289 (B-52).

Tells about care in and atmosphere of this terminal care facility. Relates poignant stories and incidents about patients and families. Emphasizes importance of facilitating communication, maintaining patient with pain relief. Twenty-two photographs.

307. ______ . "St. Christopher's Hospice," in *Death: Current Perspectives*, pp. 516-523 (B-56).
Section of the Hospice's 1971-72 Annual Report. Discusses historical origins of hospice tradition; comments on the workings of St. Christopher's including information about inquiries received, patients admitted, and composition of staff. Notes teaching, clinical studies, and research activities undertaken. Two patients' stories illustrate St. Christopher's aims.

308. ______ . "Care of the Dying. A Death in the Family: A Professional View." *British Medical Journal*, 1: 30-31, January 6, 1973.
Printed version of speech given at symposium on "Care of the Dying." Comments on what was learned from patients, importance of relieving pain and involving of entire family in patient's care.

309. SCHOENBERG, Bernard. "The Nurse's Education for Death," in *Death and Bereavement*, edited by Austin H. Kutscher. Springfield, Ill.: Charles C Thomas, Publisher, 1969. Pp. 55-74.
Consultant psychiatrist discusses use of group conferences to help students cope with crises of dying, death. Many observations regarding nursing education no longer applicable, but two reports of nursing students' work with dying patients are pertinent.

310. ______ . "Management of the Dying Patient," in *Loss and Grief*, pp. 238-260 (B-51).
Discusses importance of physician establishing, maintaining patient's trust, communicating with him about his situation, respecting his defenses, providing hope. Comments on patient and staff needs for psychiatric consultation. Illustrates value of psychotherapy for dying patients with case report. Discusses euthanasia.

311. SCHOENBERG, Bernard and Arthur C. Carr. "Psychosocial Aspects of Oral Care in the Dying Patient," in *The Terminal Patient: Oral Care*, pp. 3-15 (B-39).
Highlights problems relating to oral care management of the dying patient with case summary of Sigmund Freud. Comments on

changing attitudes toward dying patients and death and indicates why oral care is "one of the greatest challenges" in care of dying.

312. SCHOENBERG, Bernard and Robert A. Senescu. "The Patient's Reaction to Fatal Illness," in *Loss and Grief*, pp. 221-237 (B-51).
Comments on problems involved and factors to consider in providing care to persons viewed as dying. Considers pain and guilt, dependency, anger, loss of self-esteem, loss of pleasure, reactions to surgery. Gives examples of patients' responses.

313. SCHOWALTER, John E. "The Child's Reaction to His Own Terminal Illness," in *Loss and Grief*, pp. 51-69 (B-51).
Indicates child's responses to dying/impending death are influenced by his understanding of death and reactions of those around him. Identifies, discusses, and gives clinical examples to illustrate how differing responses relate to developmental stages.

314. ______ . "Anticipatory Grief and Going on the 'Danger List,' " in *Anticipatory Grief*, pp. 187-192 (B-53).
Believes this official designation that hospitals use for critically or terminally ill patients is psychologically harmful to patients. Discusses reactions of patients, parents, staff, and other child patients to an individual's placement on the danger list on pediactric ward.

315. ______ . "Drugs, Fatally Ill Children and the Pediatric Staff," in *Psychopharmacologic Agents for the Terminally Ill and Bereaved*, pp. 296-306 (B-26).
Discusses the difficulties professionals experience in caring for dying children. Comments on drugs usually prescribed for keeping child comfortable, and emphasizes that a child's emotional set is determined by the psychodynamic meanings of his condition and his relationship to parents and staff, and that his "*experience of physical discomfort* is greatly influenced by the emotional set."

316. ______ . "Pediatric Nurses Dream of Death," in *The Nurse as Caregiver for the Terminal Patient and His Family*, pp. 147-150 (B-12).
Discusses the difficulties nurses experience in caring for dying children and ways nurses can help themselves to cope better in work with these children. Discusses how dreams were used as helping tool and provides typical dream examples.

317. SCHWAB, Sister M. Loyola. "The Nurse's Role in Assisting Families of Dying Geriatric Patients to Manage Grief and Guilt," in *ANA Clinical Sessions: American Nurses' Association, 1968 Dallas*. New York: Appleton-Century-Crofts, 1968. Pp. 110-116.

Discusses importance of understanding grieving process in work with families of dying older persons; interplay of grief and guilt. Three clinical situations illustrate how nursing intervention incorporating grief process enables nurse to provide objective, nonjudgmental support to family.

318. SEITZ, Pauline M. "The Deadborn Infant: Supportive Care for Parents," in *The Nurse as Caregiver for the Terminal Patient and His Family*, pp. 104-113. (B-12).

Discusses the impact of fetal death on parents and hospital staff and factors to consider in giving parents the option of seeing the dead infant. Excerpts from a process recording illustrate the therapeutic way in which a mother was assisted in reaching her decision.

319. SEITZ, Pauline M. and Louise H. Warrick. "Perinatal Death: The Grieving Mother." *American Journal of Nursing*, 74: 2028-2033, November 1974. Also in *Dying and Grief: Nursing Interventions,* pp. 137-147 (B-45).

Nurses use Kubler-Ross's stages of dying as guidelines for work with mothers in antepartum clinic when fetal death occurs. Article considers neonates who are not expected to live and effect of mother-child contact until child's death. Discusses anxiety accompanying subsequent pregnancies.

320. SELDON, Elaine. ". . . even the Elderly." *RN Magazine*, 39:66,70, January, 1976.

Tells how a wife's hope, faith, and love changed attitudes of nurses toward 70-year-old patient they considered hopeless. Renewed nursing care efforts made it possible for wife to take husband home and care for him until his death.

321. SENESCU, Robert A. "The Problem of Establishing Communications with the Seriously Ill Patient." *Annals of the New York Academy of Sciences*, 164: 696-706, December 19, 1969.

Describes difficulties in bringing about and maintaining satisfactory communications. Focuses on illness reactions that determine meaningful interactions between patient and others. Explores implications of parental role that care providers may assume. Discusses importance of recognizing and meeting the pleasure needs of dying patients. Comments on patient anger and hostility; expands remarks during discussion period.

322. SHARE, Lynda. "Family Communication in the Crisis of a Child's Fatal Illness: A Literature Review and Analysis." *Omega*, 3: 187-201, August, 1972.

Considers the protective and open communication approaches. Discusses each approach in terms of a child's source of anxiety, death conceptions, and behavioral responses to illness through use of many excerpts from the literature. Cites 44 references.

323. SHARP, Donna. "Lessons from a Dying Patient." *American Journal of Nursing*, 68: 1517-1520, July, 1968.

Private duty nurse recounts changes in patient's behavior prior to and after physician's disclosure of fatal illness. Describes attempts to help patient cope with dying situations, efforts to communicate with hospital nursing staff about patient's care, distressing personal feelings experienced.

324. SHEPHARD, Melba W. "This I Believe – About Questioning the Right to Die." *Nursing Outlook*, 16: 22-25, October, 1968. Also in *The Dying Patient: A Nursing Perspective*, pp. 15-24 (B-6).

Discusses need to examine unquestioned life prolongation that brings suffering and indignity to patients. Raises questions about the alternatives, contrasting theological concepts with scientific idealogies and their effects upon attitudes toward dying and death. Companion article to Armiger, cited in Entry A-13.

325. SHEPHARDSON, Jan. "Team Approach to the Patient with Cancer." *American Journal of Nursing*, 72: 488-491, March, 1972. Also in *Nursing and the Cancer Patient*, pp. 38-46 (B-7).

Notes benefits of team method. Considers communication problems most persistent difficulty in care of patients with cancer. Describes how team conferences help find effective nursing care approaches. Comments on problems staff face regarding life prolongation, pain control, lifesaving efforts.

326. SHUSTERMAN, Lisa R. "Death and Dying: A Critical Review of the Literature." *Nursing Outlook*, 21: 465-471, July, 1973. Also in *Dying and Grief: Nursing Interventions*, pp. 207-221 (B-45).

A survey (not very critical) of research projects primarily concerned with the experience of dying in modern general hospitals and reactions of staff to dying patients and death. Focuses on techniques used in collecting data. Cites 45 references.

327. SIBBERS, Frances V. "Thursday Afternoon at Lunch." *American Journal of Nursing*, 74: 1308-1309, July, 1974. Also in *Dying and Grief: Nursing Interventions*, pp. 60-62 (B-45).

On last day of clinical experience, four nursing students share their perceptions of the impersonal, insensitive attitudes of staff nurses toward dying patients and wonder whether "we will get like that?"

328. SIMMONS, Sandra and Barbara Given. "Nursing Care of the Terminal Patient." *Omega*, 3: 217-225, August, 1972.

Nurses report interview study of 51 hospitalized patients to find out whether they would talk about their diagnoses, dying, or death if given opportunities. Examples of patients' conversation and accounts of patient-personnel interaction included. Discusses need for planned conversation and listening time; how information is misinterpreted; implications for nursing action in assigning personnel, working with families, dealing with patients' loneliness and hope.

329. SIMMS, Lillian M. "Dignified Death: A Right Not a Privilege." *Journal of Gerontological Nursing*, 1: 21-25, November/December, 1975.

Comments on dying of institutionalized aged persons noting how attitudes and behaviors of nursing and medical staff, as well as their educational backgrounds, are contributing factors to patients' undignified death.

330. SINGLETARY, Yvonne. "Case Report," in *The Nurse as Caregiver for the Terminal Patient and His Family*, pp. 74-82 (B-12).

When a 50-year-old man is told truth about his advanced cancer, he is given an opportunity to work through some of his unresolved conflicts with the assistance of a hospital liaison nurse, who talks with him daily until his death.

331. SMART, Ninian. "Philosophical Concepts of Death," in *Man's Concern with Death*, pp. 25-35 (B-63).

Essay distinguishes death from dying; dying with awareness from dying without awareness. Discusses emotions experienced when facing death; how facing fact of imminent death differs from process of dying.

332. SMITH, Ann G. and Lois T. Schneider. "The Dying Child: Helping the Family Cope with Impending Death." *Clinical Pediatrics*, 8: 131-134, March, 1969.

Outlines child's concept of death; uses clinical examples to illustrate children's reactions to dying. Describes some parents' reactions to their dying child; comments on value of their participation in child's care.

333. SMITH, David H. "Some Ethical Considerations in Caring for the Dying," in *ANA Clinical Sessions: American Nurses' Association, 1974 San Francisco*. New York: Appleton-Century-Crofts, 1975. Pp. 177-183.

Explores issue of mercy killing by criticizing both the "participant" viewpoint, which advocates patient rights, and the "administrative" viewpoint, with its bias toward same treatment for all and efficient use of resources. Argues that neither view is adequate and suggests factors needed to determine more appropriate criteria.

334. SOBEL, David E. "Death and Dying." *American Journal of Nursing*, 74: 98-99, January, 1974.

Series of statements suggesting fear in dying relates to dread of losing affection of loved one before death, not to death itself.

335. SOLNIT, Albert J. "Annotations: The Dying Child." *Developmental Medicine and Child Neurology*, 7: 693-695, December, 1965.

Comments on literature about subject; need for a rationale in helping dying child and family cope with dying process which involves denial, anticipatory mourning, many levels of truth. Notes need to assure child of pain relief, of not being completely alone.

336. SOLNIT, Albert J. and Morris Green. "Psychologic Considerations in the Management of Deaths on Pediatric Hospital Services: I. The Doctor and the Child's Family." *Pediatrics*, 24: 106-112, July, 1959.

Discusses factors for physician to consider and his responsibility in preparing parents before child's death. Outlines steps for informing parents and siblings of child's death. Suggests ways to help family after the death, with emphasis on importance of listening. Comments on physician's reactions to child's death.

337. ______ . "The Pediatric Management of the Dying Child: Part II. The Child's Reaction to the Fear of Dying," in *Modern Perspectives in Child Development*, edited by Albert J. Solnit and Sally A. Provence. New York: International Universities Press, 1963. Pp. 217-228.

Describes developmental concepts of death and emphasizes need to understand them in order to help child cope with impending death. Identifies child's needs; uses care provided four-year-old boy to illustrate how needs are met. Describes effects of an 11-year-old's knowledge of her impending death on parents and staff. Gives other examples of children's reactions. Advocates openness between dying child, family, and physician.

338. SONSTEGARD, Lois and others. "Dealing with Death; The Grieving Nurse." *American Journal of Nursing*, 76: 1490-1492, September, 1976. Also in *Death and Grief: Nursing Interventions*, pp. 43-47 (B-45).

Describes measures a nursing administration implemented to provide support to nursing staff caring for dying patients. Shows how nurses caring for the dying move through Kubler-Ross' stages of dying.

339. SPEER, Gertrude M. "Learning about Death." *Perspectives in Psychiatric Care*, 12, no. 2:70-73, 1974.

Nurse transferred to medical-surgical nursing unit after 20 years of psychiatric nursing elects to work with dying patients and tells how planned half-hour daily visits with three patients affected them.

340. SPITZER, Stephan P. and Jeanette R. Folta. "Death in the Hospital: A Problem for Study." *Nursing Forum*, 3, no. 4: 85-92, 1964.

Reports effects of expected and unexpected death upon one hospital's communication system. Little disruption follows expected death and standard communication patterns are used; examples show difference when unexpected death occurs.

341. STANTON, Gilbert. "Nutritional Care of the Dying Patient," in *Oral Care of the Aging and Dying Patient*, pp. 111-121 (B-38). Also in *Oral Care of the Aging and Dying Patient*, edited by Austin H. Kutscher and Ivan K. Goldberg. Springfield, IL: Charles C Thomas, 1973, pp. 111-121.

Views feeding as a major problem that may have fundamental significance in eliminating many of the intercurrent problems associated with dying patient's illness. Discusses various means for providing nourishment with aim of establishing the greatest degree of comfort.

342. STEELE, Shirley. "Nursing Care of the Child with Terminal Illness," in *Nursing Care of the Child with Long-Term Illness*, edited by Shirley Steele. New York: Appleton-Century-Crofts, 1971. Pp. 547-583.

Focuses on reactions of nursing students to dying children. Presents review of literature; comments on home care; discusses nursing contributions possible in outpatient clinic situations; considers specific nursing interventions for hospitalized child's care. Includes list of care ideas and case report with study questions. Cites 39 references. Updated version of publication in press.

343. STEWART, Barbara M. "Living with Cancer." *Nursing Forum*, 13, no. 1: 52-58, 1974.

Nurse working with predominently black and Spanish-speaking cancer clients describes how she focused on activating each patient's human potential to formulate a pattern of living with cancer rather than patterning a course of dying.

344. STORLIE, Frances. "Gloria." *American Journal of Nursing* 75: 1188-1190, July, 1975. Also in *Dying and Grief: Nursing Interventions*, pp. 55-59 (B-45).

During nurse-friend's funeral, author recalls their conversations and the poignant moments they spent together before friend's death.

345. STRAUSS, Anselm L. "Awareness of Dying," in *Death and Dying*, pp. 108-132 (B-47).

Reprint of part of Chapter One, which considers the overall problem of awareness of dying, and all of Chapter Three, which focuses on closed awareness, from *Awareness of Dying* (B-23).

346. ______ . "Family and Staff During Last Weeks and Days of Terminal Illness." *Annals of the New York Academy of Sciences*, 164: 687-695, December 19, 1969.

Discusses the complex juggling of tasks, people, and relationships that are required to prevent disruption of work and mood when patient is dying. Describes the problems presence of the dying patient's family poses for staff and the activities involved when preparing family for death. Discussed in greater detail in chapter eight of the book *Time for Dying* (B-24).

347. STRAUSS, Anselm L. and Barney Glaser. "Awareness of Dying," in *Loss and Grief*, pp. 298-309 (B-51).

Discusses how people's unwillingness to talk of dying and death influences dying persons and the hospital care situation. Outlines conditions contributing to closed awareness and the consequences of this, especially for nurses. Describes mutual pretense and the complexity of open awareness.

348. ______ . "Patterns of Dying," in *The Dying Patient*, pp. 129-155 (B-5).

Condenses research results from *Time for Dying* (B-24), which describes the different modes and courses of dying on different types of hospital wards. Explains dying trajectories and the sentimental mood which influences patient care. Includes recommendations for improving the care of dying patients.

349. STRAUSS, Anselm L., Barney G. Glaser, and Jeanne C. Quint. "The Nonaccountability of Terminal Care." *Hospitals*, 38:73-87, January 16, 1964.

Observes that nursing and medical personnel are not held accountable for the social and psychological aspects of a patient's care and indicates the consequences this has for terminally ill patients, their families, and the hospital staff. Discusses need to determine what requires accountability and the problems involved in making such requirements.

350. SUDNOW, David. "Dying in a Public Hospital," in *The Dying Patient*, pp. 191-208 (B-5).

Contrasts biological with social death, using vivid examples of hospital personnel and others who acted as though living patients were already dead. Notes how hospital redefines facts of death in terms of its own needs. Identifies factors conditioning ways dying persons and death are viewed. Contrasts the organization values of public hospitals with private ones.

351. Task force on Death and Dying of the Institute of Society, Ethics, and the Life Sciences. "Refinements in Criteria for the Determination of Death: An Appraisal." *Journal of the American Medical Association*, 221:48-53, July 3, 1972.

Report unanimously agreed upon, after 18 months deliberation, by biologists, lawyers, laymen, philosophers, physicians, social scientists, and theologians. Discusses philosophical, linguistic, medical, legal, and other death concerns with which group struggled. Lists eight characteristics necessary for "good criteria of death," including "Criteria of the Ad Hoc Committee of the Harvard Medical School," and evaluates them.

352. TAYBACK, Matthew. "Death with Dignity." *Journal of Gerontological Nursing*, 1:42-44, July/August, 1975.

Comments on factors influencing care of dying persons 65 and older, who constitute over 70 percent of the deaths reported annually in the United States, and on legislation for death with dignity.

353. TOCH, Rudolph. "Too Young to Die," in *Psychosocial Aspects of Terminal Care*, pp. 65-76 (B-52).

Views childhood death as "classic tragedy with every member of the cast playing a well-defined role." Outlines roles in considering responses of children from birth to five; six to ten; ten through adolescence. Discusses needs of parents; how siblings are affected.

354. UFEMA, Joy K. "Dare to Care for the Dying." *American Journal of Nursing*, 76: 89-90, January, 1976. Also in *Dying and Grief: Nursing Interventions*, pp. 1-3 (B-45).

Staff nurse tells of pride and personal satisfaction derived from work with dying patients and their families.

355. VEATCH, Robert M. "Choosing Not to Prolong Dying." *Medical Dimensions*, 11:8-10+ December, 1972.

Comments on chaos technological advances create in care of the dying. Discusses: confusion regarding euthanasia and need to distinguish between killing and omitting or stopping treatment; use of ordinary and extraordinary means; prolonging living and prolonging dying. Emphasizes rights of patients regarding treatments and decisions. Raises questions about establishing policies related to life prolongation choices and about legislation permitting death with dignity.

356. VERNICK, Joel and Myron Karon. "Who's Afraid of Death on a Leukemia Ward?" *American Journal of Diseases of Children*, 109: 393-397, May, 1965.

"Everyone – and the resolution of this fear is everyone's problem." Describes study of 51 hospitalized children at National Cancer Institute using "life space" interviews and weekly parent meetings. Examples show advantages of sharing knowledge of diagnosis with child and disadvantages of protection and evasion.

357. VERWOERDT, Adriaan. "Communicating with the Fatally Ill." *CA – A Cancer Journal for Clinicians,* 15:105-111, March, 1965. Available from American Cancer Society.

Comments on communication problems between physicians and patients with cancer, identifies the complex factors and considderations involved in informing patients of their prognoses. Notes factors that threaten the relationship and proposes helpful techniques physicians can use to reduce the threat.

358. VERWOERDT, Adriaan and Ruby Wilson. "Communication with Fatally Ill Patients: Tacit or Explicit?" *American Journal of Nursing*, 67: 2307-2309, November, 1967. Also in *The Dying Patient: A Nursing Perspective*, pp. 89-94 (B-6).

Says providing effective nursing care requires nurse to have clear information about what patient knows of his condition; identifies factors that serve as cues in assessing a patient's awareness of his situation. Discusses signals patients send and advantages of tacit communication.

359. VISPO, Raul H. "Critique of 'Denial and Depression.' " *Psychiatric Quarterly*, 45, no. 3: 405-409, 1971.

Summarizes impression of Abrams' article cited in Entry A-3. Comments on her use of imprecise terms and demonstrates how the clinical example used does not substantiate author's claims.

360. WAECHTER, Eugenia H. "Children's Awareness of Fatal Illness." *American Journal of Nursing*, 71:1168-1172, June,

1971. Also in *The Dying Patient: A Nursing Perspective*, pp. 215-223 (B-6).

Nurse describes study to measure anxiety scores in four groups, age six to ten. Children with fatal illness had scores twice as high as other groups. Reports how aware child is about his situation and how unaware his parents believe him to be. Provides several stories to illustrate children's awareness.

361. WAGNER, Berniece M. "Teaching Students to Work with the Dying." *American Journal of Nursing*, 64: 128-131, November, 1964. Also in *The Dying Patient: A Nursing Perspective*, pp. 201-213 (B-6).

Describes efforts of university faculty to teach care of terminally ill. Excerpts from students' papers illustrate how assigned readings related to nursing and how they facilitated discussion of practical and philosophical problems.

362. WALD, Florence S. "Development of an Interdisciplinary Team to Care for Dying Patients and Their Families," in *ANA Clinical Conferences: American Nurses' Association, 1969 Minneapolis/ Atlanta.* New York: Appleton-Century-Crofts, 1970. Pp. 47-55.

Describes physical facilities and care provided patients/families at St. Christopher's Hospice, and brief staff nurse experience that stimulated desire to create similar facility in United States. Compares care of dying in England and United States. Describes launching exploratory interdisciplinary study of dying patients and their families.

363. WALKER, Margaret. "The Last Hour Before Death." *American Journal of Nursing*, 73:1592-1593, September, 1973.

Nurse reports on a "dramatic last-hour experience with a 70-year-old 'apparently well' heart patient" who, "knowing" she was about to die, requested her son's presence at the hospital.

364. WANGENSTEEN, Owen H. "Unconditionally Yes," in *Should the Patient Know the Truth*? pp. 72-78 (B-58).

Physician says keeping truth from patient is violation of trust. Gives positive clinical examples as rationale for truth telling, cites negative consequences of deception.

365. WATSON, M. Jean. "Death – A Necessary Concern for Nurses." *Nursing Outlook*, 16: 47-48, February, 1968. Also in *The Dying Patient: A Nursing Perspective*, pp. 196-200 (B-6).

Indicates why nursing students need to understand reality of death. Outlines content and teaching methods used in incorporating subject into nursing course.

366. "A Way of Dying." *Atlantic Monthly*, 199: 53-55, January, 1957. Also in *Social Interaction and Patient Care*, edited by James K. Skipper, Jr. and Robert C. Leonard. Philadelphia: J. B. Lippincott, 1965. Pp. 179-184.

Widow describes feelings of anguish, grief, anger, and helplessness when unable to stop intervention that prevented hospitalized husband from dying in peace and dignity; how medical orientation of nursing and medical staff determined their actions despite imminence of death and wishes of patient and family.

367. WEBER, Leonard J. "Ethics and Euthanasia: Another View." *American Journal of Nursing*, 73: 1228-1231, July, 1973. Also in *Dying and Grief: Nursing Interventions*, pp. 74-80 (B-45).

Responds to Fletcher's moral defense of authanasia (Entry A-104). Argues against active authanasia as a violation against the person. Views decision not to resuscitate as "fully compatible with respect for the fullness of human meaning."

368. WEISMAN, Avery D. "Misgivings and Misconceptions in the Psychiatric Care of Terminal Patients." *Psychiatry*, 33, no. 1: 67-80, 1970.

Comments on physicians' lack of educational preparation for dealing with psychological, environmental, and emotional factors related to dying and death, and on their generally negative attitudes. Discusses ways their death attitudes influence behavior of those around dying patients. Views death as as interpersonal crisis and medical fact. Describes bereavement of the dying and the defenses professionals use. Discusses how ten general misconceptions about dying affect patient care.

369. ______ . "Psychosocial Considerations in Terminal Care," in *Psychosocial Aspects of Terminal Care*, pp. 162-172 (B-52).

Identifies three stages of fatal illness; focuses on symptom relief and safe conduct goals of medical care. Believes "adequate relief of pain is mandatory" and discusses ways of preventing or controlling "secondary suffering." Gives clinical examples to illustrate levels of denial and different kinds of anxiety dying person experience.

370. WEISMAN, Avery D. and Thomas P. Hackett. "Predilection to Death." *Psychosomatic Medicine,* 23, no. 3:232-256, 1961. Also in *Death and Identity*, pp. 293-329 (B-20). Also in *Death and Identity*, revised edition, pp. 288-317 (B-21).

Presents and discusses five reports of "predilected" patients. Evaluates care of dying patients in general. Defines and comments on impersonal, interpersonal, intrapersonal, and subjective death. Discusses appropriate death and requirements for facilitating, planning, and implementing psychotherapeutic intervention with patients certain to die.

371. WENTZEL, Kenneth B. "The Dying Are the Living." *American Journal of Nursing*, 76:956-957, June, 1976.

Chaplain gives impression of St. Christopher's Hospice where leave-taking at death is unrushed, tearful. Discusses beliefs that serve as guiding principles in providing care: that "dying patients need more attention" and that they should be allowed "as much control over their daily affairs as is possible."

372. WHITE, Joanne. "Yes, I Hear You, Mr. H." *American Journal of Nursing*, 75: 411-413, March, 1975.

Nurse recounts experiences with dying, hospitalized 77-year-old. Focuses on lung cancer symptomatology, nursing care based on Maslow's need theory; gives examples of interpersonal exchanges.

373. WHITMAN, Helen H. and Shelby J. Lukes. "Behavior Modification for Terminally Ill Patients." *American Journal of Nursing*, 75: 98-101, January, 1975. Also in *Dying and Grief: Nursing Interventions*, pp. 4-10 (B-45).

Offers do's, don'ts, and principles for altering maladaptive behavior in dying patients. Describes intervention with two patients who do not die. Conveys condescending "nurse knows best" attitude.

374. WIENER, Jerry M. "Reaction of the Family to the Fatal Illness of a Child," in *Loss and Grief*, pp. 87-101 (B-51).

Discusses impact child's illness and death has on family and coping mechanisms employed. Considers need, option, and right of parents to participate in treatment of hospitalized child and process of anticipatory grief. Indicates factors influencing impact of dying and death situation on siblings. Makes suggestions for physicians which have implications for other health care personnel involved with dying child and his family.

375. ______ . "Response of Medical Personnel to the Fatal Illness of a child," in *Loss and Grief*, pp. 102-115 (B-51).

Discusses factors contributing to reactions health care personnel – particularly in nursing and medicine – may experience in careing for dying children. Indicates need for personnel's awareness of their own attitudes and values regarding dying and death; stresses need for effective communication among all team members to facilitate care. Reports findings of survey that assessed pediatrician's attitudes and practices in care of dying children.

376. WILLIAMS, Shirley L. "The Nurse as Crisis Intervener," in *The Nurse as Caregiver for the Terminal Patient and His Family*, pp. 33-49 (B-12).

Identifies three areas in which nurses can play a major role in work with dying patients. Discusses ten categories of patients' problems and indicates how they can serve as assessment guides during interviews and guide the nurse "to facilitate supporting, comforting interventions within the patient's own value system." Cites 17 references.

377. WISE, Doreen J. "Learning About Dying." *Nursing Outlook*, 22: 42-44, January, 1974. Also in *Dying and Grief: Nursing Interventions*, pp. 176-180 (B-45).

Nurse-teacher incorporates three-phase death and dying unit into course dealing with cultural response to death and grieving. Discusses identification of one's own response; specific nursing interventions. Comments on use of simulated interaction.

378. WOEHNING, Marilee and Ida M. Martinson. "Family Nursing During Death and Dying," in *Contemporary Community Nurs-*

ing, edited by Barbara W. Spradley. Boston: Little, Brown and Company, 1975. Pp. 405-411.

Using Lindemann's stages of grief, provides clinical vignettes. Discusses family's tasks: caring for dying member; dealing with life-death paradox; expressing grief; relinquishing the person; dealing with variant roles; adjusting to external institutions.

379. WOLFF, Ilse S. "The Magnificence of Understanding," in *Should the Patient Know the Truth?*" pp. 29-39 (B-58).

Points out that truth telling is not an either-or issue. Views the problem in terms of ethical concepts and interdisciplinary relationships and nurses's own feelings regarding fatal prognoses.

380. WYGANT, W. E. Jr. "Dying, But Not Alone," *American Journal of Nursing*, 67: 574-577, March, 1967. Also in *The Dying Patient: A Nursing Perspective*, pp. 95-102 (B-6).

Hospital chaplain discusses various behaviors dying persons and family members display when facing impending death. Describes supportive intervention in work with 32-year-old woman, her 35-year-old husband, and their two children.

381. YATES, Susan A. "Stillbirth: What a Staff Nurse Can Do." *American Journal of Nursing*, 72: 1592-1594, September, 1972. Also in *Contemporary Nursing Series. Maternal and Newborn Care: Nursing Interventions*, compiled by Mary H. Browning and Edith P. Lewis. New York: American Journal of Nursing Company, 1973. Pp. 108-111.

Nurse clinician interviews mothers and learns which actions and responses of nurses were helpful to them in dealing with loss of an infant. Provides cues for action in planning care for grieving parents.

382. YEAWORTH, Rosalee C., Fredric T. Kapp, and Carolyn Winget. "Attitudes of Nursing Students Toward the Dying Patient." *Nursing Research*, 23: 20-24, January/February, 1974. Also in *Dying and Grief: Nursing Interventions*, pp. 189-198 (B-45).

Findings in questionnaire survey of 108 freshman and 69 senior nursing students to measure attitudes towards death and dying reveals senior students were more accepting of feelings, more open in communication, and had greater flexibility in relating to dying patient and their families than freshman; suggests attitude shifts that can result from nursing education.

section B
books

Section B consists of annotations of books, including collections of original papers or previously published articles. Some selections from the collections are annotated as individual entries in Section A. The annotations in Section B alert the reader to these items by giving the name of the author, the title, and the Section A entry number where the annotation can be found. For papers now in reprint collections, the Section A citation usually gives information on the original source of the reprint.

section B books

1. AGEE, James. *A Death in the Family.* New York: Bantam Books, 1971 [1938]. 318 pp.

   Deeply moving account of tragic, sudden death of young, healthy father of two small children. Focuses principally on feelings and reactions of the wife as news of her husband's fate is awaited with hope and dread during the hours immediately preceding and following knowledge of his death. Story evokes emotional responses that facilitate an understanding of shock, disbelief, grief, and other distresses that accompany experience of sudden death of a loved one.

2. AMERICAN Friends Service Committee. *Who Shall Live? Man's Control over Birth and Death. A Report Prepared for the American Friends Service Committee.* New York: Hill and Wang, 1970. 144 pp.

   Chapter Four of this volume considers population problems, control over birth, quality of life, and religious and ethical issues; focuses on man's control over death. Considers changes related to increased life expectancy, effect of medical advances on prolonging life of dying patients, and ethical implications involved in medical decisions. Comments on revised definitions of death, euthanasia, and social effects of a prolonged life span. Raises many questions.

3. BEAUVOIR, Simone de. *A Very Easy Death.* Translated by Patrick O'Brian. New York: G. P. Putnam's Sons, 1966. 106 pp. Paper edition, Warner Books, 1973.

   Author describes own feelings, thoughts, reactions, and behavior during the several months of her mother's erratic and difficult course of dying and at her death from cancer. Shares impressions of institutional care and attitudes and actions of physicians, nurses, and others involved with care, and indicates how these affected self, sister, and mother. Discusses misgivings about allowing surgical intervention without mother's consent or knowledge; evasion tactics used by self, sister, physicians, nurses, and others to protect mother from knowledge of fatal situation; discovery of written note after death of mother indicating she knew she was dying.

4. BOWERS, Margaretta K., Edgar N. Jackson, James A. Knight, and Lawrence LeShan. *Counseling the Dying.* New York: Jason Aronson, 1975. 183 pp.

   Psychiatrist, clergyman, educator, and psychologist draw on

their experiences in discussing problems encountered in work with dying persons. Authors incorporate observations and studies of others in descriptions of how death is met by dying persons and those about them, how dying persons pose threat for physicians and clergy, and how these professionals wear "masks" when talking with dying persons. Book gives rationale for psychotherapy with terminally ill persons and stresses therapy goals that help patients live until they die. Elaborates on moral and ethical issues involved in being truthful with the dying, examines common difficulties in communication between care providers and dying persons, and offers suggestions for promoting more effective communication. Ten-page bibliography.

5. BRIM, Orville G. Jr., Howard E. Freeman, Sol Levine, and Norman A. Scotch, editors. *The Dying Patient*. New York: Russell Sage Foundation, 1970. 390 pp.

Introduction by the editors. The 14 articles in this volume attempt to clarify the many problems dying and death pose for individuals, families, health professionals, and society in general. Book is divided into three sections: The Social Context of Dying; How Doctors, Nurses, and Hospitals Cope with Death; Termination of Life – Social, Ethical, Legal, and Economic Questions. A concluding chapter deals with dying as a field of research. The following contributions are annotated in Section A of this bibliography:

Glaser, Robert J. Innovations and heroic acts in prolonging life, A-123.

Knutson, Andie L. Cultural beliefs on life and death, A-195.

Kubler-Ross, Elisabeth. The dying patient's point of view, A-205.

Lasagna, Louis. Physicians' behavior toward the dying patient, A-220. The prognosis of death, A-221.

Levine, Sol and Norman A. Scotch. Dying as an emerging social problem, A-225.

Rabin, David L. with Laurel H. Rabin. Consequences of death for physicians, nurses, and hospitals, A-290.

Strauss, Anselm L. and Barney G. Glaser. Patterns of dying, A-348.

Sudnow, David. Dying in a public hospital, A-350.

The book concludes with a 63-page, briefly annotated bibliography on death and dying compiled by Richard A. Kalish.

6. BROWNING, Mary H. and Edith P. Lewis, compilers. *The Dying Patient: A Nursing Perspective*. Contemporary Nursing Series. New York: The American Journal of Nursing Company, 1972. 275 pp.

Contains 37 articles on death and dying published between January, 1962, and May, 1972, in the *American Journal of Nursing, Nursing Outlook,* and *Nursing Research.* Articles annotated in Section A of this bibliography are:

Armiger, Sister Bernadette. Reprise and dialogue, A-13.

Baker, Joan M. and Karen C. Sorensen. A patient's concern with death, A-23.

Blewett, Laura J. To die at home, A-43.

Bonine,Gladys N. Students' reactions to children's deaths, A-45.

Braverman, Shirley J. Death of a monster, A-49.

Bright, Florence and Sr. M. Luciana France. The nurse and the terminally ill child, A-51.

Burnside, Irene M. You will cope, of course, A-57

Davidson, Ramona P. Lets talk about death: to give care in terminal illness, A-76.

Death in the first person (Anonymous), A-78.

Eisman, Roberta. Why did Joc die? A-90.

Engel, George L. Grief and grieving, A-95.

Geis, Dorothy P. Mothers' perceptions of care given their dying children, A-117.

Glaser, Barney G. and Anselm L. Strauss. The social loss of dying patients, A-120.

Goldfogel, Lenda. Working with the parent of a dying child, A-125.

Hoffman, Esther. Don't give up on me! A-166.

Kneisl, Carol R. Thoughtful care for the dying, A-191.

Kubler-Ross, Elisabeth. What is it like to be dying? A-206.

McDonald, Molly. Farewell to a friend, A-234.

McNulty, Barbara J. St. Christopher's outpatients, A-236.

Maxwell, Sister Marie. A terminally ill adolescent and her family, A-248.

Mead, Margaret. The right to die, A-249.

Mervyn, Frances. The plight of dying patients in hospitals, A-251.

Quint, Jeanne C. Awareness of death and the nurse's composure, A-284. Obstacles to helping the dying, A-285.

Quint, Jeanne C. and Anselm L. Strauss. Nursing students, assignments, and dying patients, A-289.

Saunders, Cicely. The last stages of life, A-303.

Shepard, Melba W. This I believe – about questioning the right to die, A-324.

Verwoerdt, Adriaan and Ruby Wilson. Communications with fatally ill patients: tacit or explicit? A-358.

Waechter, Eugenia H. Children's awareness of fatal illness, A-360.

Wagner, Berniece M. Teaching students to work with the dying, A-361.

Watson, M. Jean. Death–a necessary concern for nurses, A-365.

Wygant, W. E., Jr. Dying, but not alone, A-380.

The remaining reprints, which are not annotated in this bibliography, are:

Jourard, Sidney M. Suicide: an invitation to die.

Levine, Myra E. Benoni.

Robinson, Alice M. What man shall live and not see death?

Vaillot, Sister Madeleine. Hope: the restoration of being.

Vanden Bergh, Richard L. Lets talk about death: to overcome inhibiting emotions.

7. BROWNING, Mary H. and Edith P. Lewis, compilers. *Nursing and the Cancer Patient*. Contemporary Nursing Series. New York: The American Journal of Nursing Company, 1973. 354 pp.

Forty-one articles published in the *American Journal of Nursing, Nursing Outlook,* and *Nursing Research* are reprinted in this volume and grouped within the following sections: Nursing Approaches; Emotional and Phychological Aspects; Current Treatment; Head and Neck Cancer; Intestinal and Urinary Diversion; and Cancer of the Breast. The following articles are annotated in Section A of this bibliography:

Barckley, Virginia. Enough time for good nursing, A-25. The crises in cancer, A-26.

Craytor, Josephine. Talking with persons who have cancer, A-74.

Fox, Jean E. Reflections on cancer nursing, A-108.

Klagsbrun, Samuel C. Communication in the treatment of cancer, A-186.

Knox, Merrily F. . . . And the cells grow, A-193.
Meinhart, Noreen T. The cancer patient: living in the here and now, A-250.
Quint, Jeanne C. The impact of mastectomy, A-282.
Shepardson, Jan. Team approach to the patient with cancer, A-325.

The remaining reprints in this publication are not listed here because they are not pertinent to the theme of this bibliography.

8. CAUGHILL, Rita E., editor. *The Dying Patient: A Supportive Approach.* Boston: Little, Brown and Company, 1976. 228 pp. Consists of seven original articles and one that has been revised and reprinted. Each selection is annotated in Section A of this bibliography.

Assell, Ruth A. If you were dying. . ., A-18.
Caughill, Rita E. Coping with death in acute care units, A-65.
Supportive care and the age of the dying patient, A-66.
Elder, Ruth G. Dying and society, A-92.
Gartner, Claudine R. Growing up to dying: the child, the parents, and the nurse, A-116.
Green-Epner, Carol S. The dying child, A-133.
Hopkins, Clark. The right to die with dignity, A-169.
Kneisl, Carol R. Grieving: a response to loss, A-192.

9. COOK, Sarah S. *Children and Dying: An Exploration and a Selective Bibliography.* Second edition. New York: Health Sciences Publishing Corporation, 1974. 106 pp.

A collection of 14 essays written by various authors and grouped under section headings titled: How Children Feel and React to Death; How Adults React to the Sick, Dying, or Bereaved Child; and Working Constructively with the Dying or Bereaved Child.

Reprinted from the first edition are Cook's "Children's Perceptions of Death," in which she uses many references and quoted passages from reported studies and observations in discussing implications for nursing in work with dying children (the article has 52 footnotes and a bibliography with 58 citations); Edgar N. Jackson's "Helping Children Cope with Death" and "Understanding the Teenager's Response to Death"; and Domeena C. Renshaw's "The Dying Child," which outlines differences between dying children and adults.

Among the pertinent essays in this second edition are Dalia Keyser's "Tears and Protest: A Mothers's Remembrances," excerpted from her book-length manuscript about her adolescent son who died of leukemia, and Elizabeth F. Young's "Explaining Death to Young Children: A Discussion of Concepts and a Bibliography," which has 44 briefly annotated citations. The book contains no index.

10. CURTIN, Leah. *The Mask of Euthanasia*. Cincinnati: Nurses Concerned for Life, 1976. 68 pp.

Nurse author describes her concern about euthanasia for newborn, mentally ill, aged, and dying persons. Excerpts from reports of action taken to cause death presented to stimulate questions and discussion of ethical, legal, moral, and medical issues involved in current proposal for the legislation of euthanasia. Publisher's address: Nurses Concerned for Life, 3400 Lehman Road, Cincinnati, OH 45205.

11. DAVIDSON, Barbara K. *You Didn't Know My Father. A Play on Death with Dignity*. New York: Family Service Association of America, 1973. 22 pp. Note: For information about having a professional cast present this half-hour drama, write Plays for Living, Family Service Association of America, 44 East 23 Street, New York, NY 10010.

Relatives talk with one another outside intensive care unit while waiting to hear about or see their particular loved one who may be dying. Terminally ill persons are a teenage son, an elderly father, and a comatose mother. Interactions poignantly portray impact of illness and impending death on patients, family members. Adult children of aging father learn of his living will and express their feelings about respecting it. Play ends with silence as code for unit is called.

12. EARLE, Ann M., Nina T. Argondizzo, and Austin H. Kutscher, editors. *The Nurse as Caregiver for the Terminal Patient and His Family*. New York: Columbia University Press, 1976. 252 pp.

Consists of 22 papers selected from those presented at a thanatology symposium on the role of the nurse in the care of the dying patient and the bereaved. Selections annotated in Section A of this bibliography are:

Benoliel, Jeanne Quint. Overview: care, cure, and the challenge of choice, A-38. Death influence in clinical practice: a course outline for the nursing school curriculum, A-37.

Coyne, A. Barbara. The nurse's responsibilities, A-72.

Eaton, James S., Jr. Coping with staff grief, A-89.

Greenleaf, Nancy P. Stereotyped sex-role ranking of caregivers and quality care for dying patients, A-134.

Kovacs, Liberty. A personal perspective of death and dying, A-199.

Lowenberg, June S. Working through feelings around death, A-231.

Schowalter, John E. Pediatric nurses dream of death, A-316.

Seitz, Pauline M. The deadborn infant: supportive care for the parents, A-318.

Singletary, Yvonne. Case report, A-330.

Williams, Shirley L. The nurse as crisis intervener, A-376.

The remaining papers (which are not annotated in this bibliography) are:

Chandler, Kenneth A. Continuing and discontinuing care.

Fennelly, Joseph F. Female chauvinism in nursing.

Fineman, Beverly C. Teaching to individual differences.

Friedenberg, Eleanor C. Continuing education in aging and long-term care.

Jacobi, Eileen M. Nursing and the therapeutic relationship.

Liaschenko, Joan M. and Richard Torpie. A case review on death, from two perspectives.

Koestenbaum, Peter. The existential meaning of death.

Proulx, Joseph R. Let the teacher beware!

Rogers, Joy and M. L. S. Vachon. Therapeutic intervention with the bereaved.

Vachon, M. L. S., W. A. L. Lyall and J. Rogers. The nurse in thanatology: what she can learn from the woman's liberation movement.

Warren, Lucy. The terminally ill child, his parents.

13. EASSON, William M. *The Dying Child: The Management of the Child or Adolescent Who Is Dying.* Springfield, Il: Charles C Thomas, Publisher, 1970. 103 pp.

Considers how developmental stages and age influence the understanding of and reaction to personal death. Discusses aspects of death to which dying children and adolescents react. Comments on disease symptoms, treatment procedures, diagnosis and prognosis, hospitalization, changes in the patient and in his role relationships, and physiological death. Uses separate chapters to elaborate on emotional development and maturational tasks of the child from birth through his fifth year, the grade-school child, and the adolescent. Points out behavioral differences seen in young adolescents (10 to 15), older adolescents, and young adults, in their attitudes toward death and reactions to dying situations. Clinical examples are not given and suggestions for working with each age group are generalized. Reactions of the dying child's family to the problems with which they are confronted, and their feelings of blame, guilt, and anger are considered. The final chapter focuses on health care personnel and provides a general discussion on the treating staff's involvement with dying children, adolescents, and their families, and on how the staff's reactions and responses affect care and treatment.

14. EPSTEIN, Charlotte. *Nursing the Dying Patient: Learning Processes for Interaction*. Englewood Cliffs, NJ: Prentice-Hall, 1975. 210 pp.

Presents individual/group games and exercises and simulated care situations designed to help health care workers acquire a repertoire of interaction skills that can enhance their communication with the dying. Separate chapters provide the framework for proposed learning activities and are based on sketchily outlined concepts related to stages of dying, dying trajectories, levels of awareness, and care of dying children, adults, and aged persons.

15. EUTHANASIA Educational Council. *Dilemmas of Euthanasia.* Excerpts from papers and discussion at the Fourth Euthanasia Conference, New York Academy of Medicine, December 4, 1971. New York: The Council, 1971. 42 pp. Available from The Euthanasia Educational Council.

Excerpts of speeches by lawyer, physician, and nurse who discuss, respectively, legal dilemmas and dilemmas facing physicians and nurses in their work with patients. Discussion moderated by Joseph Fletcher. Includes letter from clergyman supporting euthanasia based on his experience in nursing home both as clergyman and patient.

16. EUTHANASIA Educational Council. *Euthanasia Rights and Realities.* Excerpts from papers and discussion at the Fifth Euthanasia Conference, New York Academy of Medicine, December 2, 1972. New York: The Council, 1972. 48 pp.

Available from The Euthanasia Educational Council.

Physician says conflict about direct and indirect euthanasia centers on "the definition of man as a person; the dimensions of trust." Proposes third alternative, which perceives euthanasia as "permission to die, given to those overburdened by disease or age." Medical director comments on patterns of dying, social circumstances of death, and the need to redefine concepts of dignity in dying. Lawyer cites and discusses court cases involving rights of families who refused treatment or were forced to accept it. Pediatric nurse describes special problems in care of dying children and in allowing them to die.

17. EUTHANASIA Educational Council. *Death and Decisions*. Excerpts from papers and discussion at the Seventh Annual Euthanasia Conference, New York City, December 7, 1974. New York: The Council, 1974. 30 pp. Available from The Euthanasia Educational Council.

Joseph Fletcher uses eight-rung ladder symbol to depict placement of attitudes toward euthanasia, with the lowest rung representing the anti-euthanasia position. Argues that active and passive euthanasia are different procedurally, but that the two types are ethically and morally the same. Physician counters Fletcher's argument by placing the absolute anti-euthanasia position on the highest rung of the ladder to demonstrate the view that "life is the highest good." Another discussant says active and passive euthanasia are, and should remain, separate entities; argues against active euthanasia; believes physicians can align themselves with passive form only – rungs two to five on Fletcher's ladder.

18. EUTHANASIA Educational Council. *Changing Attitudes Toward Euthanasia*. Excerpts from papers presented at the Eighth Annual Euthanasia Conference, New York City, December 6, 1975. The Council, 1975. 30 pp. Available from The Euthanasia Educational Council.

Psychiatrist suggests why physicians have greater problems with euthanasia issue than other professional groups; takes a pro-euthanasia position. Lawyer explains why right to die and euthanasia movement must be integral part of the patients' rights movement; believes changes in attitude toward the rights of patients, not legislation, is the vital factor. Legislator discusses opposition encountered in efforts to introduce bill giving patient the right to decide about his life and dying. Swiss physician tells how acts of omission in care of chronically ill dying patients resulted in his arrest and indictment for murder.

19. FEIFEL, Herman, editor. *The Meaning of Death*. New York: McGraw-Hill Book Company, 1959. 351 pp. Paperback edition, McGraw-Hill Paperbacks, 1965.

A collection of 19 original and reprinted articles are assembled in this classic book. Contributions are grouped under the following five section titles: Theoretical Outlooks on Death; Developmental Orientation Toward Death; Death Concepts in Cultural and Religious Fields; Clinical and Experimental Studies; and Discussion. The following selections are annotated in Section A of this bibliography:

Aronson, Gerald J. Treatment of the dying person, A-15.
Hutschnecker, Arnold A. Personality factors in dying patients, A-171.
Kasper, August M. The doctor and death, A-181.
Nagy, Maria H. The child's view of death, A-260.

The following articles are not annotated in this bibliography.

Hoffman, Frederick J. Grace, violence and self. Reprinted as: Mortality and modern literature.
Jung, Carl G. The soul and death.
Richter, Curt P. The phenomenon of unexplained sudden death in animals and man.
Wahl, Charles W. The fear of death.

20. FULTON, Robert, editor. *Death and Identity*. New York: John Wiley & Sons, 1965. 415 pp.

Editorial comments introduce the four sections of this collection of 28 reprints. The sections are titled: Theoretical Discussions on Death; Attitudes and Responses Toward Death; Grief and Mourning–The Reaction to Death; Ceremony, the Self, and Society. Reprints annotated in Section A of this bibliography are:

*Lindemann, Erich. Symtomatology and management of acute grief, A-228.
Natterson, Joseph M. and Alfred G. Knudson, Jr. Oberservations concerning fear of death in fatally ill children and their mothers, A-262.

*Weisman, Avery D. and Thomas P. Hackett. Predilection to death, A-370.

The other articles are listed below in alphabetical sequence by author:

*Alexander, Irving E. and Arthur M. Adlerstein. Affective responses to the concept of death in a population of children and early adolescents.

*Alexander, Irving E., and Randolph S. Colley, and Arthur M. Adlerstein. Is death a matter of indifference?

Barry, Herbert, Jr. Significance of maternal bereavement before age of eight in psychiatric patients.

Borkenau, Franz. The concept of death.

Brewster, Henry H. Separation reaction in psychosomatic disease and neurosis.

Christ, Adolph E. Attitudes toward death among a group of acute geriatric psychiatric patients.

Diggory, James C. and Doreen Z. Rothman. Values destroyed by death.

Feifel, Herman. Attitudes of mentally ill patients toward death

*Fulton, Robert. The sacred and the secular: attitudes of the American public toward death, funerals, and funeral directors.

Fulton, Robert and Gilbert Geis. Death and social values.

*Hilgard, Josephine R., Martha F. Newman, and Fern Fisk. Strength of adult ego following childhood bereavement.

Jeffers, Frances C., Claude R. Nichols, and Carl Eisdorfer. Attitudes of older persons toward death.

Kalish, Richard A. Some variables in death attitudes.

*Lifton, Robert J. Psychological effects of the atomic bomb in Hiroshima: the theme of death.

*Mandelbaum, David G. Social uses of funeral rites.

Paz, Octavio. The day of the dead.

*Rhudick, Paul J. and Andrew S. Dibner. Age, personality, and health correlates of death concerns in normal aged individuals.

*Shoor, Mervyn and Mary H. Speed. Death, delinquency, and the mourning process.

Shrut, Samuel D. Attitudes toward old age and death.

Stern, Karl, Gwendolyn M. Williams, and Miguel Prados. Grief reactions in later life.

*Swenson, Wendell M. Attitudes toward death among the aged.

Teicher, Joseph D. "Combat fatigue" or death anxiety neurosis.
*Volkart, Edmund H. and Stanley T. Michael. Bereavement and mental health.
Wahl, Charles W. The fear of death.
*Warner, W. Lloyd. The city of the dead.

Also contains a 17-page bibliography.

*These items can also be found in the revised edition of this book, cited in Entry B-21.

21. FULTON, Robert, and Robert Bendiksen, editors. *Death and Identity,* Revised edition. Bowie, MD: The Charles Press, 1976. 448 pp.

Fourteen articles that appeared in the first edition of this book (see Entry B-20) have been replaced by newer selections. Editorial comments are in keeping with the changes. An index has been added and the bibliography has been reduced to eight pages. Among the new selections, Robert Fulton and Julie Fulton's "A Psychosocial Aspect of Terminal Care: Anticipatory Grief," is annotated in Entry A-112 of this bibliography. The Contributions by Erich Lindemann, Avery D. Weisman, and Thomas P. Hackett Cited in Entry B-20 are retained. Not annotated in this bibliography are:

Bendiksen, Robert. The sociology of death.
Bendiksen, Robert and Robert Fulton. Death and the child: an anterospective test of the childhood bereavement and later behavior disorder hypothesis.
Berardo, Felix. Widowhood status in the United States: perspective on a neglected aspect of the family life cycle.
Blauner, Robert. Death and social structure.
Clayton, Paula, Lynn Desmarais, and George Winokur. A study of normal bereavement.
Feifel, Herman. Religious conviction and fear of death among the healthy and the terminally ill.
Glaser, Barney G. and Anselm L. Strauss. Awareness contexts and social interaction.
Lifton, Robert J. The sense of immortality: on death and the continuity of life.
Parsons, Talcott, Renee C. Fox, and Victor M. Lidz. The gift of life and its reciprocation.
Pine, Vanderlyn R. and Derek L. Phillips. The cost of dying: a sociological analysis of funeral expenditures.

Schulz, Richard and David Aderman. Effect of residential change on the temporal distance to death of terminal cancer patients.

Sudnow, David. Dead on arrival.

Templer, Donald I. The construction and validation of a death anxiety scale.

22. FULTON, Robert, Jerry Carlson, Karl Krohn, Eric Markusen, and Gregg Owen, compilers. *Death, Grief, and Bereavement: A Bibliography, 1845-1975.* New York: Arno Press, 1977. 258 pp.

Entries are listed alphabetically by author and numbered consecutively to total 3, 806 citations. A subject index facilitates access to the entries.

23. GLASER, Barney G. and Anselm L. Strauss. *Awareness of Dying.* Chicago: Aldine Publishing Company, 1965. 305 pp.

Presents a theory of awareness based on extensive field research and interviews which examine the behavior of dying patients and those about them. Examines expectation of death as a problem of social definition and as a way of determining how much an individual knows, or ought to know, about his dying situation. Separate chapters define, explore, and illustrate situations and circumstances that contribute to closed awareness, suspicion awareness, mutual pretense, open awareness, and discounting awareness. Problems of awareness are discussed and presented in relation to: direct disclosure of terminality; the unaware family; the aware family; and the "nothing-more-to do" phase and its effect upon a nurse's composure. Considers the practical use of awareness theory.

24. ______ . *Time for Dying.* Chicago: Aldine Publishing Company, 1968. 270 pp.

Companion to *Awareness of Dying* cited in Entry B-23. Authors view dying as a temporal process and examine the temporal features of dying in hospitals. Book describes and discusses how differing organizational structures of wards affect the behavior of staff, patients, families; ways in which the organization of hospital does or does not fit into an individual patient's course of dying or dying trajectory. Separate chapters explain how initial trajectories are determined and examine the lingering trajectory, the expected and unexpected quick dying trajectories and trajectory endings.

Final chapter makes recommendations for improving care of the dying.

25. GLASSER, Ronald J. *Ward 402.* New York: George Braziller, 1973. 232 pp. Paperback edition, Pocket Books, 1974.

Physician uses novel as vehicle to describe experiences while an intern on a pediatric unit of large teaching hospital. Tells how involvement with dying 11-year-old girl and her parents helped him discover that the practice of medicine consists of more than treating a case, body part, or disease. Moving narrative and outspoken dialogue indicate growing awareness that medical care must include concern for and understanding of the person who has the disease, and consideration of feelings, needs, and rights of parents, including the right to refuse life-prolonging measures. Though characters and events are fictionalized, recorded incidents are true in essence.

26. GOLDBERG, Ivan K., Sidney Malitz, and Austin H. Kutscher, editors. *Psychopharmacologic Agents for the Terminally Ill and Bereaved.* New York: The Foundation of Thanatology, 1973. 339 pp.

Thirty-five selected papers prepared by a multidisciplinary health professional group for the purpose of disseminating information about the problems inherent in treatment with psychopharmacologic agents and how their knowledgeable and specific use affects the various approaches to the general care of the dying and bereaved. The following contributions are annotated in Section A of this bibliography:

Bader, Madelaine A. Personalizing the mangement of pain for the terminally ill patient, A-21.

Buschman, Penelope R., Sarah L. Sheets, and Ann Wharton. Use of psychopharmacologic agents in the care of the terminally ill child, A-58.

Klerman, Gerald L. Drugs and the dying patient, A-187.

Kubler-Ross, Elisabeth. On the use of psychopharmcologic agents for the dying patient and the bereaved, A-212.

Malitz, Sidney and Eda G. Goldstein. Psychotherapy and pharmacotherapy in a dying patient: report of a supervised case, A-241.

Schowalter, John E. Drugs, fatally ill children, and the pediatric staff, A-315.

27. GROLLMAN, Earl A., editor. *Explaining Death to Children*. Boston: Beacon Press, 1967. 296 pp.

An anthology presenting a blend of information and perspectives from the fields of religion, psychology, psychiatry, sociology, anthropology, biology, and children's literature that can expand and clarify an adult's understanding of both children and death. The following contributions are annotated in Section A of this bibliography:

Grollman, Earl A. Prologue: explaining death to children, A-136.

Kastenbaum, Robert. The child's understanding of death: how does it develop? A-182.

Rochlin, Gregory; How younger children view death and themselves, A-297.

28. ____. *Concerning Death: A Practical Guide for the Living*. Boston: Beacon Press, 1974. 365 pp.

A question-and-answer book in which knowledgeable professionals give answers to questions about 20 areas of concern related to preparing for death, death, and the aftermath of death to facilitate understanding and to serve as a guide for persons affected by dying and death. Answers relate to questions about: care of the dying patient; children and death; physicians' involvement with the fatally ill and their families; Jewish, Protestant, and Roman Catholic ways of death and mourning; funeral and burial arrangements; insurance and legal details; and correct social behavior with the bereaved.

29. GROLLMAN, Earl A. *Talking about Death: A Dialogue Between Parent and Child*. Revised edition. Boston: Beacon Press, 1976. 98 pp.

The purpose of this book is to help parents explain the meaning and reality of death to children. Designed to be used over time and read aloud to a child, a parent's guide for facilitating explanations accompanies the page or pages the parent selects to read. A listing of agencies and organizations that can provide parents with further help is given, and suggestions are offered for further reading, listening, and viewing.

30. GUNTHER, John. *Death Be Not Proud: A Memoir.* Memorial edition. New York: Harper & Row Publishers, 1971 [1949]. 295 pp.

Author relates story of son's valiant and courageous 15-month struggle with illness and relentlessly progressing brain tumor. Depicts supportive, loving relationships between son and self and son and his mother that helped sustain patient's hope. Describes shattering effect knowledge of fatal diagnosis had on both parents, their responses to the situation, their frantic search for ways to stay the fatal outcome, and their efforts to protect their son from knowledge of his impending death. This edition contains excerpts and letters written by the boy, entries from his diary, a reaction written by his mother, and a new introduction.

31. HAMOVITCH, Maurice B. *The Parent and the Fatally Ill Child.* Duarte, CA: City of Hope Medical Center, 1964. 152 pp.

Reports findings of research program conducted at City of Hope Medical Center where parents actively participated in care of their dying children; discusses benefits for parents, children, and involved personnel. Sample case of three-year-old boy includes report of staff observations, staff meetings, and follow-up interview with parents after child's death.

32. HINTON, John. *Dying.* Second edition. Baltimore: Penguin Books, 1972. 220 pp.

Focuses on the dying individual, the persons about him, and those who will grieve at his death. Discusses fatal illnesses; problems related to evaluating and alleviating pain and relieving other distressing physical symptoms. Elaborates on factors influencing a patient's anxieties, fears, and emotional state. Emphasizes need to care for the whole person and to provide support for the dying patient's relatives and friends. Notes the value of nursing care. Indicates complexities involved in talking with patients about their condition and assessing how much they want to know. Examines issues of prolonging life and/or hastening death; advantages and disadvantages of caring for dying persons at home; and problems inherent in caring for them in acute hospital settings. Concludes with discussion of bereavement reactions, mourning, and restitution.

33. KASTENBAUM, Robert and Ruth Aisenberg. *The Psychology of Death.* New York: Springer Publishing Company, 1972. 498 pp. Paperback edition (shortened version), 1976.

An abundantly referenced publication that examines and integrates what has been learned about man's relationship to death and the ways in which our actions are affected by our ideas and attitudes about death. The scope is broad, and includes discussion about death as a thought, psychological factors in death and longevity, and suicide and murder. Emphasis is upon the clinical and theoretical contributions made by behavioral and social scientists. Historical sources are incorporated and speculation is made about the future. The ninth chapter examines the cultural milieu of death today and focuses discussion on the "professionals in our death systems," namely, the funeral director, physician, nurse, clergyman, and mental health specialist. A useful resource book.

34. KRANT, Melvin J. *Dying and Dignity: The Meaning and Control of a Personal Death.* Springfield, Il: Charles C Thomas, Publisher, 1974. 154 pp.

Written to help individuals, families, and health care professionals "look at some of the tribulations that beset us all and ask if there is a way to enhance the sense of dignity and control all of us need throughout life." Focuses on the nature of the dying experience for persons with a fatal illness. Discusses some facts about dying today, fears regarding death, and the indignities of dying. Views dying principally as a medical problem and elaborates upon euthanasia as peaceful death. Considers the problems, perceptions, and interactions of families in regard to fatal illness, and makes some proposals for education of health professionals.

35. KUBLER-ROSS, Elisabeth. *On Death and Dying.* New York: The Macmillan Company, 1969. 260 pp. Paperback edition, 1970. 284 pp.

General comments on societal influences and attitudes about death and dying in the United States, followed by description of author's work with over 200 dying patients that led to observation that the dying process involves five identifiable stages – anger, denial, bargaining, depression, and acceptence – each of which is defined, described, and illustrated with case reports and dialogues with dying patients. Stresses importance of providing patients with hope, suggests actions that can convey hope, and uses a transcribed interview to illustrate the phenomenon of everpresent hope. Discusses disruptive effect a patient's illness and dying has on his family and the problems involved in communication between and among patient, family, and hospital staff. Presents transcribed interviews with four patients to give a picture of each patient's awareness, problems, concerns, and wishes, and to illustrate the variety of responses and reactions of both patients and interviewer. Discusses how patients, in contrast to hospital staff, responded positively to death and dying seminars; how physicians were most resistive and nurses least so; and how, as objections gradually diminished, care of dying patients improved. Eleven-page bibliography.

36. ______ . *Questions and Answers on Death and Dying*. New York: Macmillan Publishing Company, 1974. 192 pp. Paperback edition, Collier Books, 1974.

Questions most frequently asked of the author in workshops, lectures, and seminars on the care of dying patients are grouped under the following chapter headings and answered: The Dying Patient; Special Forms of Communication; Suicide and Terminal Illness; Sudden Death; Prolongation of Life; Where Do We Best Care for Our Dying Patients?; The Family's Problems after Death has Occurred; Funerals; Family and Staff Deal with Their Own Feelings; Other Staff Problems; Old Age; Questions of Humor and Fear, Faith, and Hope; Personal Questions.

37. ________ , editor. *Death: The Final Stage of Growth*. Human Development Books: A Series in Applied Behavioral Science. Englewood Cliffs, NJ: Prentice-Hall, 1975. 181 pp. Paperback edition, 1975.

Kubler-Ross introduces 15 essays by various authors who present different religious, cultural, philosophical, and personal viewpoints on dying and death. Summarizes what she herself learned from her years of work with dying patients. The contributions are grouped into the following sections: Why Is It so Hard to Die?; Death Through Some Other Windows; Dying Is Easy, but Living Is Hard; Death and Growth: Unlikely Partners?; Death: The Final Stage of Growth. The following contributions are annotated in Section A of this bibliography:

Carey, Raymond G. Living until death, A-59.
Death in the first person (Anonymous), A-78.
Imara, Mwalimu. Dying as the last stage of growth, A-172.
Kubler-Ross, Elisabeth. Death as part of my own personal life, A-214.

Mauksch, Hans O. The organizational context of dying, A-247.
Pitkin, Dorothy. One woman's death – a victory and a triumph, A-277.

38. Kubler-Ross, Elisabeth. *Images of Growth and Death* (Prentice-Hall) and *On Children and Death* (Macmillan).

The Prentice-Hall publication is listed in *Books in Print 1976*, but the book will not be published. In the introduction to her book, *Questions and Answers on Death and Dying*, Kubler-Ross refers to a forthcoming book titled *On Children and Death*. This book was not published as of June, 1977.

39. KUTSCHER, Austin H., Bernard Schoenberg, and Arthur C. Carr, editors. *The Terminal Patient: Oral Care*. New York: The Foundation of Thanatology, 1973. 272 pp.

Twenty-six papers selected from those presented at a symposium on the significance of oral care for the terminally ill and dying patient are grouped under these headings: Selected Medical Specialties; Dentistry; Nursing; Social Work; and Pastoral Care. Annotated in Section A of this bibliography are:

Bader, Madelaine A. Nursing care and interpersonal relationships, A-20.
Schoenberg, Bernard and Arthur C. Carr. Psychosocial aspects of oral care in the dying patient, A-311.

40. KUTSCHER, Martin L., Daniel J. Cherico, Austin H. Kutscher, Amy E. Hanninen, Stephen Johnson, and David Peretz. *A Comprehensive Bibliography of the Thantology Literature*. New York: MSS Information Corporation. 1975. 285 pp.

Total of 4,844 numbered citations listed by author. Contains a 40-page subject index to facilitate use.

41. LUND, Doris. *Eric*. Philadelphia: J. B. Lippincott Company, 1974. 345 pp. Paperback edition, Dell Publishing Company, 1975. 267 pp.

A mother's account of her son's five-year-struggle against leukemia, discovered at age 17, and his heroic fight to live a full, normal existence to the time of his death. Tells of the impact of diagnosis upon the family and of her profound feelings ranging from extreme hope to deep despair. For Mrs. Lund's story on cassette with filmstrip, see Entry C-10C.

42. MANNES, Marya. *Last Rights.* New York: William Morrow & Company, 1974. 150 pp. Signet Paperback, 1975.

Distinguished author uses word pictures and vignettes of situations involving the dying, conversations with physicians, nurses, and others involved with the dying, and excerpts from the literature and the mass media to present an argument for euthanasia. Comments on advanced medical technology that can keep a human body alive but that prolongs a person's dying, not living. Believes each person should have the right to choose the manner of his dying – in dignity.

43. NATIONAL Institute of Child Health and Human Development. *Sudden Infant Death Syndrome: Selected Annotated Bibliography, 1960-1971.* No. (NIH) 73-237. Washington, DC: U.S. Government Printing Office, 1973. 58 pp. The 239 annotated citations are grouped by year.

44. NEALE, Robert E. *The Art of Dying.* New York: Harper & Row, Publishers, 1973. 158 pp.

A series of mental exercises constructed by clergyman-author and designed to help the reader face his own death with a sense of ease rather than fear or panic. Ideas based on: decade of experience in seminars and workshops with people of all ages, backgrounds, and vocations; work with dying and bereaved persons; and personal experience of own brother's dying and death. Objective is to assist both laymen and professionals to an understanding of death as a part of life.

45. O'CONNOR, Andrea B., compiler. *Dying and Grief: Nursing Interventions.* Contemporary Nursing Series. New York: American Journal of Nursing Company, 1976. 221 pp.

Contains 33 articles published in *The American Journal of Nursing, Nursing Outlook,* and *Nursing Research* between 1973 and 1976. The following articles are annotated in Section A of this bibliography:

Andrews, Linda. The last night, A-10.

Breuer, Judith. Sharing a tragedy, A-50.

Bunch, Barbara and Donna Zahra. Dealing with death: the unlearned role, A-55.

Craven, Joan and Florence S. Wald. Hospice care for dying patients, A-73.

Fletcher, Joseph. Ethics and euthanasia, A-104.
Griffin, Jerry J. Family decision: a crucial factor in terminating life, A-135.
Gyulay, Jo-Eileen. The forgotten grievers, A-139.
Hampe, Sandra O. Needs of the grieving spouse in a hospital setting, A-146.
Hardgrove, Carol and Louise H. Warrick. How should we tell the children? A-149.
Hiscoe, Susan. The awesome decision, A-165.
Human, Mildred E. Death of a neighbor, A-170.
Ingles, Thelma. St. Christopher's Hospice, A-173.
Kobrzycki, Paula. Dying with dignity at home, A-196.
Marks, Mary J. The grieving patient and his family, A-243.
Northrup, Fran C. The dying child, A-266.
Palen, Charity S. The passage, A-275.
Robinson, Lisa. We have no dying patients, A-295.
Seitz, Pauline M. and Louise H. Warrick. Perinatal death: the grieving mother, A-319.
Shusterman, Lisa R. Death and dying: a critical review of the literature, A-326.
Sibbers, Frances V. Thursday afternoon at lunch, A-327.
Sonstegard, Lois, Neva Hansen, Linda Zillman and Mary K. Johnston. Dealing with death: the grieving nurse, A-338.
Storlie, Frances. Gloria, A-344.
Ufema, Joy K. Dare to care for the dying, A-354.
Weber, Leonard J. Ethics and euthanasia: another view, A-367.
Whitman, Helen H. and Shelly J. Lukes. Behavior modification for terminally ill patients, A-373.
Wise, Doreen J. Learning about dying, A-377.
Yeaworth, Rosalee C., Frederic T. Kapp, and Carolyn Winget. Attitudes of nursing students toward the dying patient, A-382.

Reprints that have not been annotated in this bibliography are:

Jackson, Pat L. Chronic grief.
Lester, David, Cathleen Getty, and Carol R. Kneisl. Attitudes of nursing students and nursing faculty toward death.
Miles, Helen S. and Dorothea R. Hays. Widowhood.
Zahourek, Rothlyn and Joseph S. Jensen. Grieving and the loss of the newborn.

46. PADILLA, Geraldine V., Veronica E. Baker, and Vikki A. Dolan. *Interacting with Dying Patients: An Inter-Hospital*

Nursing Research and Nursing Education Project. Duarte, CA: City of Hope National Medical Center, 1975. 219 pp.

Description of an educational program and an evaluation of its impact on nurses and the care given dying patients. Research aspects emphasized. Course materials are in appendices.

47. PEARSON, Leonard, editor. *Death and Dying: Current Issues in the Treatment of the Dying Person.* Cleveland: The Press of Case Western Reserve University, 1969.

A 102-page "Selected Bibliography on Death and Dying" by Pearson is included in the hard cover edition. The annotated citations are grouped under ten broad categories. Five eminent clinicians are the contributors to the volume. The following articles are annotated in Section A of this bibliography:

LeShan, Lawrence. Psychotherapy and the dying patient, A-222.

Saunders, Cicely. The moment of truth: care of the dying patient, A-304.

Strauss, Anselm L. Awareness of dying, A-345.

The other contributions are:

Kalish, Richard A. The effects of death upon the family.
Kastenbaum, Robert. Psychological death.

48. QUINT, Jeanne C. *The Nurse and the Dying Patient.* New York: The Macmillan Company, 1967. 307 pp.

Based on results of six-year investigation of care given by nursing and medical personnel to dying patients. Focus is on what happens to nursing students when they encounter dying patients and death. Describes and discusses how organizational and ideological conditions in the five schools of nursing studied determined how students reacted to what they were taught about care of dying patients; how they coped with dying patients and death; how teachers' attitudes and behaviors influenced the psychosocial aspects of the patients' care; and ways in which recovery care goals and lifesaving values of the nursing and hospital cultures created additional stress for students who were caring for the terminally ill and dying. Discusses the complexity of dying as a hospital event and includes students' accounts of their first encounters with death. Numerous examples of students' conversations with patients illustrate the many conversational difficulties inherent in situations related to dying and death. Comments on the consequences care by nursing students has for dying patients. Indicates nursing education programs do not have systematic approaches to problems related to dying patients and do not prepare students for the complex and serious responsibilities they will face in clinical practice. Elaborates on implications for curriculum change.

49. ROSENTHAL, Ted. *How Could I Not Be Among You?* New York: George Braziller, 1973. 77 pp.
In poetry and prose, 30-year-old author, the father of two young children, tells how learning he had leukemia and limited time to live affected him. Black and white photographs. Script for the film cited in Entry C-24.

50. RUITENBEEK, Hendrik M., editor. *The Interpretation of Death*. New York: Jason Aronson, 1973. 286 pp. Published formerly as *Death: Interpretations*. New York: Dell Publishing Company,1969. 286 pp.
Editor's essay introduces 14 reprinted materials related to dying and death, and seven that focus on mourning. The following articles are annotated in Section A of this bibliography:

LeShan, Lawrence and Eda LeShan. Psycotherapy and the patient with a limited life-span, A-224.
Norton, Janice. Treatment of a dying patient, A-267.
Rosenthal, Hattie R. Psychotherapy for the dying, A-300.

The 11 other articles on death, which are not annotated in this bibliography, are:

Cappon, Daniel. The psychology of dying.
Chadwick, Mary. Notes upon the fear of death.
Eissler, Kurt. Death and the pleasure principle.
Feifel, Herman. The problem of death.
Friedlander, Kate. On the "longing to die."
Jaques, Elliott. Death and the mid-life crises.
Jones, Ernest. On "dying together" and an unusual case of "dying together."
Rosenthal, Hattie R. The fear of death as an indispensable factor in psychotherapy.
Scher, Jordan M. Death – the giver of life.
Segal, Hanna. Fear of death.
Young, William H., Jr. Death of a patient during psychotherapy.

The seven articles on mourning are not listed here because they do not focus on the actual processes of dying and death.

51. SCHOENBERG, Bernard, Arthur C. Carr, David Peretz and Austin H. Kutscher, editors. *Loss and Grief: Psychological Management in Medical Practice*. New York: Columbia University Press, 1970. 397 pp.

Collection of 26 papers providing theoretical and practical information about man's struggle to cope with loss and grief and ways in which patients and/or family members who have experienced or anticipate loss can be assisted to accept loss. Contributions are presented in five sections and focus on the following areas of concern: phychological concepts central to loss and grief; loss and grief in childhood; reaction to and management of partial loss; the dying patient; humanistic and biologic concepts regarding loss and grief. The following selections are annotated in Section A of this bibliography:

Gonda, Thomas A. Pain and addiction in terminal illness, A-128.
Schoenberg, Bernard. Management of the dying patient, A-310.
Schoenberg, Bernard and Robert A. Senescu. The patient's reaction to fatal illness, A-312.
Schowalter, John E. The child's reaction to his own terminal illness, A-313.
Strauss, Anselm L. and Barney G. Glaser. Awareness of dying, A-347.
Wiener, Jerry M. Reaction of the family to the fatal illness of a child, A-374. Response of medical personel to the fatal illness of a child, A-375.

52. SCHOENBERG, Bernard, Arthur C. Carr, David Peretz, and Austin H. Kutscher, editors. *Psychosocial Aspects of Terminal Care*. New York: Columbia University Press, 1972. 388 pp.

Contains 27 papers selected from those presented at a symposium on care of terminally ill patients with reports of 13 workshops conducted at the conference. The following contributions are annotated in Section A of this bibliography:

Abrams, Ruth D. The responsibility of social work in terminal cancer, A-4.
Benoliel, Jeanne Quint. Nursing care for the terminal patient: a psychosocial approach, A-35.

Dobrof, Rose. Community resources and the care of the terminally ill and their families, A-80.

Fulton, Robert and Julie Fulton. Anticipatory grief: a psychosocial aspect of terminal care, A-113.

Futterman, Edward H., Irwin Hoffman and Melvin Sabshin. Parental anticipatory mourning, A-115.

Heinemann, Henry O. Human values in the medical care of the terminally ill, A-152.

Henderson, Edward. The approach to the patient with an incurable disease, A-153.

Krant, Melvin J. In the context of dying, A-201.

Kubler-Ross, Elisabeth. Hope and the dying patient. A-211.

Kutscher, Austin H. The psychosocial aspects of the oral care of the dying patient, A-217.

Maddison, David and Beverley Raphael. The family of the dying patient, A-238.

Saunders, Cicely. A therapeutic community: St. Christopher's Hospice, A-306.

Toch, Rudolf. Too young to die, A-353.

Weisman, Avery D. Psychosocial considerations in terminal care, A-369.

53. SCHOENBERG, Bernard, Arthur C. Carr, David Peretz, Austin H. Kutscher, and Ivan K. Goldberg, editors. *Anticipatory Grief*. New York: Columbia University Press, 1974. 381 pp.

The forty-one papers, which were selected from those presented at a symposium on anticipatory grief, present concepts of anticipatory grief, discuss its impact and significance for patients' families and caregivers, and examine approaches for understanding of loss from a multidisciplinary viewpoint. The following contributions are annotated in Section A of this bibliography:

Aldrich, C. Knight. Some dynamics of anticipatory grief, A-8.

Benoliel, Jeanne Quint. Anticipatory grief in physicians and nurses, A-36.

Comerford, Brenda. Parental anticipatory grief and guidelines for caregivers, A-68.

Goldstein, Eda E. and Sidney Malitz. Psychotherapy and pharmacotherapy as enablers in the anticipatory grief of a dying patient: a case study, A-127.

Schowalter, John E. Anticipatory grief and going on the "danger list," A-314.

54. SCOTT, Frances G. and Ruth M. Brewer, compilers and editors. *Confrontations of Death: A Book of Readings and Suggested Method of Instruction*. Corvallis, OR: Continuing Education Publications, 1971. 184 pp.

Contains reprinted materials intended for use in seminars on death and dying. There is a course outline in the appendix. The following selections are annotated in Section A of this bibliography:

Glaser, Barney G. and Anselm L. Strauss. Dying on time: arranging the final hours in a hospital, A-121.

Kazzaz, David S. and Raymond Vickers. Geriatric staff attitudes toward death, A-183.

Lasagna, Louis. A person's right to die, A-219.

Saunders, Cicely. The moment of truth: care of the dying person, A-304.

The eight readings from poetry and literature include all of Leo Tolstoy's *The Death of Ivan Ilych*, annotated in Entry B-62, and excerpts from Agee's *A Death in the Family*, annotated in Entry B-1.

Not annotated in this bibliography are:

Guthrie, George F. The meaning of death.

Howard, Alan and Robert A. Scott. Cultural values and attitudes toward death.

Koestenbaum, Peter. The vitality of death.

Mitford, Jessica. Fashions in funerals.

Needleman, Jacob. The moment of grief.

Nettler, Gwynn. Review essay: on death and dying.

Pine, Vanderlyn R. and Derek L. Phillips. The cost of dying: a sociological analysis of funeral expenditures.

Thurmond, Charles J. Last thoughts before drowning.

Toobert, Saul. The simulation of personal death: a T-group experience.

55. SHEPARD, Martin. *Someone You Love Is Dying: A Guide for Helping and Coping*. New York: Harmony Books, 1975. 219 pp.

Psychiatrist/author provides layman with practical information about everyday realities of dying. Discusses ways of minimizing fear of death and of telling persons they are dying. Gives general information about physiological dying responses and the management of pain. Offers suggestions for generating honest, open communication between patient and family; advocates openness and tells of its benefits. Comments on advantages of dying at home, on details of wills, insurance policies, and funerals that must be managed, and on the period of bereavement for survivors. Quotes conversations between self and dying patients to portray their feelings and perceptions and to illustrate what the dying can teach the living, including professionals.

56. SHNEIDMAN, Edwin S. *Death: Current Perspectives.* New York: Jason Aronson, 1976. 547 pp. Paperback edition, Palo Alto, CA: Mayfield Publishing Company, 1976. 547 pp.

A collection of 40 reprinted articles and excerpts from books are assembled into four sections focusing on cultural, societal, interpersonal, and personal perspectives of death. Selections annotated in Section A of this bibliography are:

Feder, Samuel L. Attitudes of patients with advanced malignancy, A-99.
Fletcher, George P. Prolonging life: some legal considerations, A-103.
Mant, A. Keith. The medical definition of death, A-242a.
Saunders, Cicely. St. Christopher's Hospice, A-307.

Also included are exerpts from books that are annotated in this section of this bibliography. The authors and their entry numbers are: Beauvoir, Simone de, B-3; Glaser, Barney and Anselm L. Strauss, B-23 and B-24; Hinton, John, B-32; Kastenbaum, Robert and Ruth Aisenberg, B-33; Kubler-Ross, Elisabeth, B-35; Heywood, Rosalind, B-63; Toynbee, Arnold, B-63; Weisman, Avery D., B-66.

Not annotated in this bibliography are:

Aries, Philippe. Forbidden death.
Baird, Jonathan. The funeral industry in Boston.
Baruch, Joel. Combat death.
Elliott, Gil. Agents of death.
Feifel, Herman. Attitudes toward death: a psychological perspective.
Fowles, John. Human dissatisfaction.
Mac. Gatch, Milton. The biblical tradition.

Goldscheider, Calvin. The mortality revolution. The social inequality of death.
Gorer, Geoffrey. The pornography of death.
Lifton, Robert Jay and Eric Olson. The nuclear age.
Matthews, W. R. Voluntary euthanasia: the ethical aspect.
Parkes, Colin M. The broken heart.
Richards, Victor. Death and Cancer.
Russell, Bertrand. Do we survive death?
Shneidman, Edwin S. The death certificate. Death work and stages of dying. Postvention and the survivor-victim.
Shaffer, Thomas L. Psychological autopsies in judical opinions.
Silverman, Phyllis R. The widow-to-widow program: and experiment in preventive intervention.
Sudnow, David. Death, uses of a corpse, and social worth.
Toynbee, Arnold. Various ways in which human beings have sought to reconcile themselves to the thought of death.
Trombley, Lauren E. A psychiatrist's response to a life-theatening illness.
Veatch, Robert M. Brain death.
Toynbee, Arnold. Various ways in which human beings have sought to reconcile themselves to the thought of death.

57. SMITH, JoAnn K. *Free Fall.* Valley Forge, PA: Judson Press, 1975. 138 pp.

Personal account of the final months of life of wife-mother-professional religious educator who tells how her struggle with pain, distressing physical symptoms, medical treatments, and progressing cancer affected her faith, personal relationships, and emotional and physical being. Raises questions and makes pertinent observations about depersonalizing hospital rules and regulations and about how the behavior of physicians, nurses, and clergymen can be hurtful or helpful to the dying person and to his significant others. Offers suggestions for improving care of dying patients.

58. STANDARD, Samuel and Helmuth Nathan, editors. *Should the Patient Know the Truth? A Response of Physicians, Nurses, Clergymen, and Lawyers.* New York: Springer Publishing Company, 1955. 160 pp.

Twenty-four practicing professionals respond to the question and express beliefs and professional opinions about what patients should be told about their disease or the gravity of their condition and prognosis. Responses annotated in Section A of this bibliography are:

Baer, Ruth F. The sick child knows, A-22.
Davidoff, Leo M. What one neurosurgeon does, A-75.
Lewis, Eloise R. and Esther K. Sump. Sympathy and objectivity in balance, A-226.
Meyer, Bernard C. What patient, what truth? A-253.
Wangensteen, Owen H. Unconditionally yes, A-364.
Wolff, Ilse S. The magnificence of understanding, A-379.

59. STRAUSS, Anselm L. and Barney G. Glaser. *Anguish: A Case History of a Dying Trajectory*. Mill Valley, CA: The Sociology Press, 1970. 193 pp.

A reconstructive review of the pertinent events occurring during the course of a patient's four-month hospitalization and ending with her death one day after surgery. The patient's experiences, described with the aid of two involved nurses, reveal the tragic story of a woman, described as demanding, selfish, controlling, ritualistic, unreasonable, and impossible to satisfy, whose behavior negatively affected a situation fraught with tension, anger, hostility, and disorganization. Tells of communication breakdown between and among patient, physicians, nurses, and others involved in care; of nursing staff's desire to get rid of patient and physician's reluctance to discharge her; of surgeon who planned drastic surgery but neglected to tell patient of postponement. Story of a patient who desperately wanted relief from pain, information about her condition, attention, and concerned care, but was met instead with anger, intolerance, avoidance, isolation, and desertion by those responsible for her care.

60. SUDNOW, David. *Passing On: The Social Organization of Dying*. Englewood Cliffs, NJ: Prentice-Hall, 1967. 176 pp.

Report on practices, procedures, and activities of hospital personnel in a large public hospital and in a private hospital of similar size where care of the dying, techniques of breaking "bad news," and the processing of dead bodies are usually incorporated into hospital routines. Discusses differences in attitudes and behavior of personnel towards the dying and dead in the two institutions.

61. *The Thanatology Library*. New York: Highly Specialized Promotions, 1976. 32 pp.

Annotated catalog of books and audiovisual materials in the field of thanatology assembled from over 100 Publishers and available for purchase from this one source: Highly Specialized Promotions, P. O. Box 989, GPO, Brooklyn, New York 11202.

62. TOLSTOI, Leo N. *The Death of Ivan Ilych*. [1886] Translated by Louise and Aylmer Maude. New York: Health Sciences Publishing Corporation, 1973. 68 pp. Also in *Confrontations of Death,* pp. 65-92 (B-54).

Description of reactions of family and acquaintances to the death of 45-year-old husband, father, and public official precedes moving account of his plight which transcends time and culture as he seeks relief from progressive discomfort and attemps to find out what is wrong. His experiences with physicians who give contradictory opinions, the reactions of his family to his deteriorating condition, and his own feelings of anger, depression, and helplessness are powerfully depicted as he realizes he is dying and struggles to cope with his worsening condition and the denial, avoidance, isolation, and conspiracy of silence created in reponse to his impending death.

63. TOYNBEE, Arnold, A. Keith Mant, Ninian Smart, John Hinton, Simon Yudkin, Eric Rhode, Rosalind Heywood, and H. H. Price. *Man's Concern with Death*. New York: McGraw-Hill Book Company, 1968. 280 pp.

Frequently cited source in which Toynbee and other contributors look at the subject of death from the viewpoint of their own specialty -- medicine, pychiatry, theology, philosophy, anthropology, literature, and psychical research. Contributions annotated in Section A of this bibliography are:

Hinton, John. The dying and the doctor, A-161.
Mant, A. Keith. The medical definition of death, A-242a.
Smart, Ninian. Philosophical concepts of death, A-331.

The other contributions, which are not annotated in this bibliography, are:

Heywood, Rosalind. Attitudes to death in the light of dreams and other out-of-the-body-experience. Death and physical research. The present position regarding the evidence of survival.

Price, H.H. What kind of next world?

Rhode, Eric. Death in twentieth-century fiction.

Smart, Ninian. Attitudes toward death in eastern religions. Death and the decline of religion in western society. Death in the Judaeo-Christian tradition. Some inadequancies of recent Christian thought about death.

Toynbee, Arnold. Changing attitudes toward death in the modern western world. Death in war. Increased longevity and the decline of infant mortality. Perspectives from time, space, and nature. The relation between life and death, living and dying. Traditional attitudes toward death.

Yudkin, Simon. Death and the young.

64. VEATCH, Robert M. *Death, Dying, and the Biological Revolution: Our Last Quest for Responsibility*. New Haven: Yale University Press, 1976. 323 pp.

Critical, well-documented review of ethical, legal, medical, social, and philosophical issues and dilemmas created by revolutionary advances in the ability to save and prolong life. Considers technical and ethical problems involved in defining death and the issues related to dying morally and choosing not to prolong dying. Elaborates on the patient's right to refuse treatment and how this is influenced by the competency or incompetency of the dying individual. Discusses the patient's right to know the truth and the rationale for truth-telling and truth-withholding. Comments on the concept of natural death and the need for a workable public policy that reduces legal ambiguities.

65. VERWOERDT, Adriaan. *Communication with the Fatally Ill*. Springfield, IL: Charles C Thomas, Publisher, 1966. 183 pp.

Based on work with patient at Duke University Medical Center. Defines fatal illness and elaborates upon the complexities involved in informing a person he has a fatal illness. Discusses communication principles and techniques that facilitate therapeutic goals which consider the physical aspects, psychological reactions, and interpersonal vicissitudes of the illness situation. Describes defense mechanisms used by patients for coping with their situation, and elaborates on emotional responses patients exhibit in reaction to knowledge of their fatal illness. Uses clinical examples to illustrate situations and makes suggestions for action that will foster effective interventions in patient care. Emphasizes the importance of communication with families; discusses the problem the dying situation creates for them; and indicates how professionals can be helpful. Considers the special problems created by fatal illness in children, and examines religious and ethical considerations regarding telling or withholding the truth and the patient's right to know.

66. WEISMAN, Avery D. *On Dying and Denying: A Psychiatric Study of Terminology.* New York: Behavioral Publications, 1972. 247 pp.

Book based on clinical material from hospitalized patients represents attempt to learn how people come to terms with imminent death, illustrates how "knowledge about death in the abstract differs from actual contact with dying people," and identfies some general principles for recognizing and dealing with persons facing impending death. Discusses common misconceptions about dying, death, and dying patient. Explains: the process, purpose, and degrees of denial; the concept of middle knowledge; the characteristics of acceptance; factors contributing to psychosocial death; and appropriate death. Documents findings with clinical illustrations drawn from interviews with people facing death from heart disease, cancer, and old age.

67. WEISMAN, Avery D. and Robert Kastenbaum. *The Psychological Autopsy: A Study of the Terminal Phase of Life. Community Mental Health Journal Monograph No. 4.* New York: Behavioral Publications, 1968. 59 pp.

Discusses findings of psychological autopsies that examined a four-stage terminal phase of life for each of 80 patients who died in a geriatric institution. Many excerpts from case materials illustrate aspects of stages explored. Notes how psychological autopsy is analogous to somatic autopsy. Indicates how care of the dying and aged patient can be improved through help of the psychological autopsy; discusses implications for its use in general hospitals and other care facilities.

68. WERTENBAKER, Lael Tucker. *Death of a Man.* New York: Random House, 1957. 181 pp. Paperback reprint, with new introduction, Beacon Press, 1974.

In describing the last months of her husband's life, author

incorporates notes written by him which describe his thoughts and feelings about, and his behavior in response to, his fatal illness and impending death. Tells of husband's insistence on knowing and coping with truth; the reluctance of physicians to tell him the truth or to accept his refusal of palliative treatment; the problems encountered in dealing with his pain and other distressing physical symptoms; the moments of anguish and joy they experienced with each other and with their children as they faced his dying and death together; and her assistance in his suicide.

69. WINTER, Arthur, editor. *The Moment of Death: A Symposium.* Springfield, IL: Charles C Thomas, Publisher, 1969. 84 pp.

Publication resulting from conference in which neuroscientist, cardiac surgeon, and medical examiner state their viewpoints, a lawyer comments on current state of law, and a professor of medicine raises questions concerning who should make decisions about moment of death. Concern focused on determination of death in relation to transplants. Includes questions addressed to and answered by speakers. Appendix contains letters of Christian Barnard, Denton Cooley, and Norman Shumway regarding determination of death for transplantation situations.

70. WOLF, Anna W. M. *Helping Your Child to Understand Death.* Revised edition. New York: Child Study Press, 1973. 64 pp.

Written for parents and "all others who care about children," this booklet considers ways of telling children about death by suggesting responses for both children's questions and those of parents about how to help children who encounter death.

71. WORCESTER, Alfred. *The Care of the Aged, the Dying, and the Dead.* Second edition. Springfield, IL: Charles C Thomas, Publisher, 1940. 77 pp.

Considered a classic by some. The first of three chapters focuses on care of the aging and the third on care of the dead. The second chapter discusses the visibly dying individual; describes signs of approaching death and various simple measures that can enhance a patient's physical comfort. Discusses importance of understanding the dying person's personality and emphasizes the "art" rather than the "science" of medicine. Opines that "instead of any progress in the art of caring for the dying, medical practice seems to have deteriorated."

section C audiovisuals

To date, no standard format has been adopted for the listing of multimedia resources. Therefore, information about the audiovisual materials annotated in this section is given as follows: title; type of material; whether the visual material is in color or in black and white (b/w); time length in minutes; year of production (when no date is available, the initials n.d. are used); whether the material is available for rental, sale, or loan; the producer's name; the name and address of the distributor; the telephone number of the distributor when available.

Distributor sources are correct as of May, 1977. The reader is reminded, however, that distributor sources are subject to change and that individual materials may be withdrawn from circulation.

The majority of the audiovisual materials are given as individual entries. Several selections, however, are part of a set or program (see Entries C-7 and C-34 for examples). For these items, the title of the program is given with the entry number and the titles and annotations of the individual parts of the program follow.

Note: All listed films are 16 mm. When a filmstrip is accompanied by a record, it is a 12-inch LP.

1. *ABC News Close-Up: The Right to Die.* Film, color, 56 minutes, 1973, rental only, Marlene Sanders. Distributed by MacMillan Films, Inc., 34 MacQuesten Parkway South, Mount Vernon, NY 10550. (914)-664-5051.

   Documentary that explores the personal, medical, ethical, and social issues surrounding dying and death. Includes face-to-face interviews with dying persons. Raises questions about the best way for families, health professionals, and the clergy to deal with the dying. Examines issues involving whether a person should be told he is dying, whether he has the right to end his own life, and whether technological life supports should be withheld to enable a person to die with dignity. Also listed as *The Right to Die.*

2. *After Our Baby Died.* Title sometimes cited for the film, *Sudden Infant Death Syndrome–After Our Baby Died.* See Entry C-45 for annotation.

3. *Care of the Patient Who Is Dying.* Filmstrip with record or audiocassette, color, 86 frames, 20 minutes, 1969, sale only. Produced and distributed by Trainex Corporation, P.O. Box 116, Garden Grove, CA 92642. Toll free: National (800) 854-2485; California, (800) 472-2479.

   Explains need for physical, emotional, and spiritual care of the hospitalizaed dying patient; illustrates ways of providing comfort. Depicts signs of approaching death; care necessary when patient becomes unresponsive; what to do when patient dies; and how to prepare body for removal to morgue.

4. *Come Take My Hand.* Film, color, 25 minutes, 1972, rental/sale, WKYC-TV, Chicago. Distributed by Films Incorporated, 1144 Wilmette Avenue, Wilmette, IL 60091.

   Depicts ways a Dominican nun at Holy Family Home helps terminal cancer patients overcome fear as death approaches by providing love and understanding as she renders nursing care. By recognizing each patient's uniqueness and humanity, she helps both patients and families to cope.

5. *A Conference on the Dying Child.* Pediatric Nursing Series. Film, videocassette, videotape, b/w, 44 minutes, 1967, rental/sale, Video Nursing. Audiocassette, 44 minutes, 1967, sale only, Video Nursing. For all sales, contact American Journal of Nursing Company, Educational Services Division, 10 Columbus

Circle, New York City, NY 10019. (212) 582-8820. For film rentals, contact American Journal of Nursing Company, Film Library, c/o Association Films, Inc., 600 Grand Avenue, Ridgefield, NJ 07657. (201) 943-8200. For videotape rentals, contact American Journal of Nursing Company, 20 North Wacker Drive, Suite 1948, Chicago, IL 60606. (312) 641-1026.

Moderated discussion among a pediatric unit head nurse, a nursing supervisor, and a nursing instructor who exchange ideas about their reactions and attitudes toward death and dying pediatric patients. Discussants share their early personal experiences with death to illustrate the child's developing concept of death; discuss ways children talk about dying and death and the feelings nurses experience in caring for dying children. Importance of hope is stressed, and the reverse involvement of parent and staff as a child nears death is noted. Ways of dealing with a child's questions about his condition are considered; discussants disagree on "telling." Comments on ways children attempt to support and protect their parents. Note: video portion is not essential.

6. *Conversation with a Dying Friend.* Audiocassette, 50 minutes, 1972. See Entry C-13 for media details.

Interview with a young woman who tells about the impact knowledge of her dying condition had on self, family, friends, and interpersonal relationships. Describes traumatizing effect of mastectomy and the terror and stress related to progression of the disease. Views the dying situation as an identity crisis and says coming to terms with death requires growth from within, although she notes how family, friends, and health professionals can help.

7. *Coping with Death and Dying: Emotional Needs of the Dying Patient and the Family.* Talks by Dr. Elisabeth Kubler-Ross. Set of five audiocassettes, 30 minutes each, 1973, sale only. Produced and distributed by Ross Medical Associates, S.C., 1825 Sylvan Court, Flossmoor, IL 60422. (312) 798-2559. Title and annotation of each tape follows.

7A. Tape One. *The Fear of Death, Introduction: The Verbal and Nonverbal Symbolical Language.*

Kubler-Ross tells how her work with dying patients began; shares experiences, personal feelings, and "gut" reactions of self and others. Relates difficulties encountered with fellow physicians and hospital staff whose fears, defenses, and negative attitudes were greater than patients'. Says fatally ill patients know they are dying; that, by perceiving death as a catastrophic force bearing down upon helpless patients, staff can better understand the languages dying persons use. Gives two clinical examples to illustrate nonverbal symbolical language used mostly by children, and explains symbolical verbal language with accounts of a dying child and an old man ready to die.

7B. Tape Two. *Stages of Dying: Denial, Pseudo-Denial, Anger.* Discusses patients' and families' responses to impending death and the problems their reactions create for those about them. Illustrates with example of woman whose denial interfered with her care and created negative responses from those responsible for her treatment. Distinguishes denial from pseudo-denial. Tells of difficulties encountered in caring for patients and family members who respond with anger, and suggests ways to assist them. Content reiterates what is said in author's writings but delivery adds poignancy to illustrations.

7C. Tape Three. *Stages of Dying: Bargaining, Depression, Acceptance or Resignation.*
Illustrates bargaining with story of woman wanting one pain-free day. Uses experience with young man who postponed talking about dying until shortly before his death to emphasize the importance of being available to a patient when he is ready to talk of impending death. Discusses reactive depression and anticipatory grief, which are difficult for patient, his family, and hospital staff. Indicates elements that contribute to a patient's reaching the stage of acceptance and shows how acceptance differs from resignation. Comments on the problems created when patient and family are at different stages.

7D. Tape Four. *Children and Death.*
Suggests that children die more easily than do adults; says three- and four-year-olds are aware of and can talk about their impending death. Comments on separation fears of children under three and mutilation fears of three-to five-year-olds. Uses clinical example to show how the concept of death matures faster in hospitalized children than in other children. Discusses importance of assisting parents to accept the impending deaths of their children. Utilizes a series of poems written by the mother of a dying four-year-old to illustrate stages parents go through

and a child's reactions to his own dying. Comments on problems generated by adults' reluctance to permit children to talk of death.

7E. Tape Five. *Sudden Death.*
Kubler-Ross and an emergency room nurse discuss problems encountered when sudden death occurs. They consider what to say to the dying patient and his family; how to handle situations involving several injured persons when one of them asks about another who is dead; how to give information to the family in person or by telephone. Discuss rationale for having a physician inform family of a patient's death; the value of crying and screaming for the bereaved, and the need to give relatives an opportunity to see the body. Indicate the need for nurses and physicians to have an opportunity to express their feelings when resuscitation efforts fail.

8. *Crib Death–A Sudden Infant Death Syndrome . . . A Documentary.* Audiocassette, 59 minutes, 1972. See Entry C-13 for media details.

Nurse Carolyn Szybist describes the syndrome, and pathologist John I. Coe gives statistics and reviews research findings of the past decade. Parents of sudden death victims describe their anguished experiences, feelings of pain and guilt, the impact of the infant's death on their lives, and how the Sudden Infant Death Foundation provided means for sharing their grief with one another.

9. *Death.* Film, b/w, 43 minutes, 1968, rental/sale, Arthur and Evelyn Barron. Distributed by Filmakers Library, Inc., 290 West End Avenue, New York City, NY 10023. (212) 877-4486.

Story of 52-year-old man dying of cancer and followed through his last days and death at Calvary Hospital. Caring atmosphere of this institution conveyed through scenes showing physician making patient rounds, friendly manner of nursing personnel, and care of patient's body after death. Interactions between staff members and patient present few opportunities for him to talk of his concerns about dying; after his death, more is learned about him from interviews with relatives.

10. *Death and Dying: Closing the Circle.* Filmstrips with audiocassettes or records, five-part program, color, 14 to 20 minutes, discussion guide, 1975, 1976, sale as a set only. Produced and

distributed by Guidance Associates, Inc., 757 Third Avenue, New York City, NY 10017. (212) 754-3700. The title and annotation for each program follows.

10A. Part I. *The Meaning of Death.* 15 minutes. 1975.
Robert J. Lifton comments on ways medical technology and emphasis on youth have contributed to denial of death in the United States. Discusses emotions survivors often experience; ways frank discussion can ease anxiety; how people experience a "sense of immortality." Concludes with an elderly woman's philosophy of life.

10B. Part II. *A Time to Mourn, a Time to Choose.* 14 minutes 1975.
Commentary on and depiction of funeral rites, burial practices, and their alternatives in various countries of the world.

10C. Part III. *Walk in the World with Me.* 20 minutes. 1975.
In photo-essay, Doris Lund tells the story of her son's five-year struggle with leukemia. Comments on the family's changing emotions, difficult decisions, and mingled hope and acceptance. See Entry B-42 for information about Ms. Lund's book, *Eric.*

10D. Part IV. *The Critically Ill Patient.* 1976.
Interview with patient dying of cardiovascular disease. Describes patient's feelings about life, death, and his family.

10E. Part V. *The Bereaved.* 1976.
Interview with parents, sister, and wife of a young cancer victim. Health care professionals discuss ways of restructuring the family after patient dies. Explores positive approach to talking about death.

11. *Death and the Child.* Audiocassette, 45 minutes, 1972. See Entry C-13 for media details.

Workshop address in which pastoral psychologist Edgar N. Jackson discusses the need for honest and open communication with children about the dying and death of a loved one. Draws from clinical experiences to illustrate how incapacitating anxieties and fears can develop when these critical events are left unexplained or unexamined and how deception, disguise, and denial create unanticipated difficulties. Focuses on constructive approaches than can be taken, resources that can be employed, and skills that can be developed by health care professionals to help children manage the crisis of death.

12. *Death and the Family: From the Caring Professions' Point of View.* Audiocassette, 30 minutes, 1972. See Entry C-13 for media details.

Symposium address given in April, 1971, by nursing professor Delphie Fredlund. Discusses the challenges dying patients present to the care-giving professions; indicates how professionals' tendency to view death as personal failure can be devastating to patients; argues that health care professionals must confront their own fears and conflicts about death if they are to help others to face dying. Says awareness of grief processes and development of a personal philosophy of death is necessary for each caregiver, and outlines steps in philosophy development. Discusses how care of dying children presents distressing challenges for nurses. Notes that children are prevented from talking about impending death and states that the public health nurse has a critical role in helping child patients and their parents to put the experience of dying into the context of life. Gives examples of interactions with children to illustrate their views on death.

13. *Death, Grief, and Bereavement.* 24 audiocassettes, from 21-59 minutes long, 1972-1975, sale only (individually or in sets) from The Charles Press Publisher, Inc., A Division of the Robert J. Brady Company, Bowie, MD 20715. Toll free: (800) 638-0220.

Tapes initially produced and distributed by the Center for Death Education and Research at the University of Minnesota. Now all tapes are distributed by The Charles Press Publishers, Inc., and new tapes are produced in association with Insight Productions and Robert Fulton, the director of the Center for Death Education and Research. The series consists of lectures, interviews, dialogues, and oral documentaries on topics related to dying and death. Written materials accompanying the tapes give profiles of the speakers, synopses of the presentations, and bibliographies. Tapes selected for annotation in this bibliography are listed alphabetically by title and can be found under the following entry numbers: C-6, 8, 11, 12, 14, 17, 20, 26, 36, 38, 40, 44, and 46.

14. *Dialogue on Death.* Audiocassette, 59 minutes, 1972. See Entry C-13 for media details.

Tape of an informal conversation with clinical psychologist

John Brantner, sociologist Robert Fulton, and Professor Robert Slater that was given as a radio broadcast by KULM, University of Minnesota Radio, in May, 1970. Participants discuss contemporary attitudes toward death and dying; examine death-denying defenses ranging from use of euphemisms to isolation of chronically ill and dying patients; talk of the influence of changing social values, secularization, the use of complex masking behaviors, and the assumption by professionals of many roles traditionally assumed by families; comment on the problems dying and death pose for health care professionals who focus on cure and view death as failure; and speak of contemporary practices regarding funeral rituals.

15. *Dialogues on Death: Preparation for Living.* Audiocassette. A title sometimes used to cite the audiocassette programs prepared by the Center for Death Education and Research at the University of Minnesota. The correct title is *Death, Grief, and Bereavement* (see Entry C-13).

16. *The Dignity of Death.* Film, color, 30 minutes, 1973, sale only, ABC Television. Sold by American Broadcasting Company Merchandising, Inc., 1330 Avenue of the Americas, New York City, NY 10019. (212) 581-7777.

Portrays St. Christopher's Hospice in London and its approaches to relieving the physical, emotional, social, and spiritual suffering of the dying. Shows the caring, peaceful mood of the hospice, where patients' unrestricted visitors include children and pet animals, and patients are encouraged to make the most of their remaining days by spending time out-of-doors, visiting their homes, and taking short vacations when medically feasible.

17. *Dr. Cicely Saunders . . . A Medical Pioneer.* Audiocassette, 39½ minutes, 1975. See Entry C-13 for media details.

Saunders tells of the origin of St. Christopher's Hospice, of its philosophy of care, and of the active treatment that focuses on the terminally ill patient's symptoms and their relief. Tells how the control and management of physical, mental, social, and spiritual pain are tailored to meet the needs of the *person* who is dying. Discusses ways families are involved in patients' care, ways patients talk about their dying, how the staff functions and communicates with patients and each other. Contrasts hospice care and treatment with that given in large medical centers, and comments on changes that are necessary to improve care of the dying.

18. *The Dying Patient–Denial.* Filmstrip with audiocassette, color, 108 frames, 15 minutes, 1976, sale only, Decision Media. Distributed by J. B. Lippincott Company, A-V Department, East Washington Square, Philadelphia, PA 19105. Toll free (national except Pennsylvania), (800) 523-2945. Pennsylvania, call collect, (215) 574-4442.

Viewer/listener is asked to put self in position of nurse at bedside of patient who has just learned he has six months to live. Dialogue between patient and nurse is supplemented by instructor's comments about dying patient's coping mechanisms, which need to be considered in responding to the patient's denial, resentment, and self-pity. Ninety-seven of the filmstrip's 108 frames consist of the patient's facial expressions. Reverse side of the audiotape is silent.

19. *The Dying Patient–Toward Acceptance.* Filmstrip with audiocassette, color, 97 frames, 15 minutes, 1976, sale only. See Entry C-18 for producer and distributor.

Viewer/listener is asked to put self in position of nurse at bedside of patient who has just learned he has six months to live. Dialogue between patient and nurse is supplemented by instructor's comments about the patient's grief, sadness, and loss, and about ways the nurse can help the patient express his feelings. All 97 of the filmstrip's frames consist only of the patient's facial expressions. Reverse side of the audiotape is silent.

20. *Facing Death with the Patient: An On-Going Contract.* Audiocassette, 30 minutes, 1972. See Entry C-13 for media details.

Symposium address given in 1971 in which physician Vincent Hunt identifies general principles found effective in working with dying patients on a personal level. Comments on the benefits of open communication, the hazards of deception, the need to maintain hope, involve the family, and be nonjudgmental. Identifies the components and characteristics of an on-going contract and shares personal feelings and reactions to dying and death, noting how his medical education has influenced him.

21. *The Family of the Dying Patient.* Audiocassette, 23 minutes, discussion guide, 1972, sale only, American Cancer Society, 777 Third Avenue, New York City, NY 10017. To purchase, contact your local American Cancer Society.

National nursing consultant Virginia Barckley discusses the concerns and problems with which families of dying patients must cope.

Notes the particular problems created when the dying person is an aged spouse, a child, or a parent with young children. Comments on the plight of men family members, who often are excluded from assisting with care, and on the negative feelings the dying person and situation can evoke in those about him. Suggests nurse actions for providing helpful supportive care.

22. *Future Unknown.* Film, b/w, 15 minutes, discussion guide, n. d., rental only. Produced and distributed by University of Pittsburgh School of Nursing Learning Research Center, 239 School of Nursing Building, 3500 Victoria St., Pittsburgh, PA 15261.

Depicts emotional trauma experienced by young woman hospitalized for recurrent malignancy who feels hospital personnel avoid talking with her and that her physician has given up hope, and who is unable to discuss her suspicions of terminality with her husband. Nurse helps patient to express feelings about dying and death and provides needed support.

23. *Gift of Life: Right to Die.* Film, b/w, 15 minutes, 1968, rental only, National Education Television. Distributed by Audio-Visual Center, Indiana University, Bloomington, IN 47401. (812) 337-2105.

Considers ethical, moral, and medical problems involved in four types of life/death decisions: organ transplants, situations involving choice to revive one patient rather than another, euthanasia, and use of brain waves to determine death.

24. *How Could I not Be Among You.* Film, color, 29 minutes, 1972, rental/sale, Thomas Reichman. Distributed by Benchmark Films, 145 Scarborough Road, Briarcliff Manor, NY 10510. (914) 762-3838.

Pictures and filmed scenes accompany voice, conversation, and poetry of Ted Rosenthal, 30, who describes his feelings, thoughts, experiences, and reactions to knowledge he has acute leukemia and limited time to live. Tells of new freedom discovered and resultant reordering of life's priorities. For text and selected still photographs from film in book form, see Entry B-49.

25. *In Search of Life After Death.* Film, Color, 24 minutes, 1976, rental/sale, Alan Landsburg. Distributed by Pyramid Films, Box 1048, Santa Monica, CA 90406.

Various people who have been successfully resuscitated by hospital teams describe their experiences on the frontiers of death.

26. *Journey to St. Christopher's: A Hospice for the Dying.* Audiocassette, 29 minutes, 1975. See Entry C-13 for media details.
A word picture in which staff and patients describe the experience and philosophy of this 54-bed institution which focuses upon providing comfort and care to patients with long-term and terminal illnesses and which served as a model of care for large hospitals and medical institutions to emulate. Depicts how patients are made to feel welcome and safe upon their admission to the facility, and how active treatment is directed towards relief of distressing physical symptoms and control of physical, mental, social, and spiritual pain. Explains how control and management of the chronic pain of terminal illness differs from the treatment of acute pain in other conditions. Notes emphasis is on enhancing the quality of a patient's remaining life but not on prolonging the dying process.

27. *Just a Little Time.* Film, color, 21 minutes, 1973, rental/sale, Barey-Callaci-Video Nursing. Distributed by the American Journal of Nursing Company (see Entry C-5 for ordering details).
Documentary that explores shared experiences, special problems, and rewards of relationship between 49-year-old dying woman and oncologic nurse specialist. Comments of Dr. Elisabeth Kubler-Ross provide additional insights.

28. *Just a Little Time.* Audiocassette with study guide, 30 minutes, 1973, sale only. See Entry C-27 for producer and Entry C-5 for ordering details.
Designed for use in conjunction with the film, *Just a Little Time* (see Entry C-27). Consists of a nursing staff conference which focuses on developing a plan of care for the dying woman-wife-mother portrayed in the film.

29. *The Lyn Helton Story.* Also titled *Soon There Will Be no More of Me* (see Entry C-42 for annotation).

30. *The Mercy Killers: A Study of Euthanasia.* Film, b/w, 30 minutes, 1969, rental/sale, BBC-TV, London. Distributed by Time-Life Mutimedia, 100 Eisenhower Drive, Paramus, NJ 07652. (201) 843-4545.

Questions on: individual's right to decide whether to live or die; legal sanctions for physicians to end life; whether killing ever is an act of "mercy." Conflicting views on these issues expressed by physicians, lawyers, clergy, and laymen through case histories and interviews. Takes no sides.

31. *Nursing Management of the Dying Patient.* Audiocassette, 21 minutes, discussion guide, 1972, sale only. Produced and distributed by the American Cancer Society, 777 Third Avenue, New York, NY 10017. To purchase, contact your local American Cancer Society.

Discusses the need for nurses to become more involved in providing physical and emotional care for hospitalized dying patients; emphasizes individualized care. Suggests nurse actions that can help communication, convey caring, and promote feelings of security. Comments on value of the nurse's presence, gifts, and rituals as reinforcing links to living. Considers the nurse's own need for support and indicates how this can be provided.

32. *Passing Quietly Through.* Film, b/w, 26 minutes, rental/sale, 1971, Dinitia McCarthy. Distributed by Grove Press, Inc., 196 West Houston Street, New York City, NY 10014. (212) 242-4900.

Bedridden, apparently dying, aging man expresses thoughts and feelings about his life and coming death to nurse who makes daily visits to his single-room apartment and urges him to seek institutional care. Depicts nurse's involvement as she shares a significant experience in her life with this man who has no other person in the world to relate to.

33. *The Patient's Right to Die.* Videotape, b/w, 60 minutes, n.d., available without charge on borrower's raw stock tape. WRAMC-TV. Walter Reed Army Medical Center, Video-Tape Library, Room 1077, Bldg. 54, Washington, D.C. 20305, (202) 576-2823.

Lecture on the moral-ethical dilemmas in today's society. Considers how long and under what circumstances life should be preserved. Distinguishes between active and passive euthanasia and discusses minimal care concepts and extraordinary therapy.

34. *Perspectives on Dying.* Filmstrip with audiocassette or record, set of six programs, color, instructor's manual, role-playing cards, personal questionnaire, supplementary text, 1973, sale

only. Produced and distributed by Concept Media, 1500 Adams Avenue, Costa Mesa, CA 92626. (714) 549-3347. Program titles and annotations follow.

34A. Program 1. *American Attitudes Toward Death and Dying.* 89 frames, 17 minutes.
Posits that the way one lives affects how one dies. Presents situations depicting how denial of death creates difficulties in interacting with dying persons; how urbanization, advances in medical science, and secularization have influenced cultural attitudes. Illustrates how the pervasive denial of death is reflected and reinforced in daily living activities of people in this culture.

34B. Program 2. *Psychological Reactions of the Dying Patient.* 123 frames, 30 minutes.
Illustrates how a patient's responses to fatal illness are influenced by his personal characteristics, the quality of his interpersonal relationships, and the nature of his illness. Discusses the coping mechanisms of denial, regression, and intellectualization. Considers and gives examples of the emotional reactions of anger, guilt, shame, grief, and depression. Notes the importance of touch.

34C. Program 3. *Hazards and Challenges in Providing Care.* 118 frames, 28 minutes.
Illustrates how nurses' expectations and interactions influence care given patients. Compares recovery-oriented care given in emergency situations with comfort care given the terminally ill. Discusses factors that contribute to expectations nurses have of themselves and their patients; problems encountered when patients do not act as expected. Depicts how closed, suspected, mutual pretense, and open awareness states influence interactions with the dying. Considers controversy regarding use of addicting drugs and decisions regarding withdrawal of life-supporting measures. Offers suggestions for helping nurses prepare for and cope with dying patients.

34D. Program 4. *Guidelines for Interacting with the Dying Person.* 86 frames, 22 minutes.
Illustrates the importance of tone and manner as well as nurse's verbalizations in interactions with three dying patients. Empha-

sizes the importance of maintaining feelings of personal dignity, fostering a sense of security, and maintaining an element of hope then indicates ways these needs can be met. Considers how to encourage patients in self-expression, and the importance of listening.

34E. Program 5. *Viewpoint: The Dying Patient.* 122 frames, 31 minutes.
Emotion-evoking presentation of two patients whose words reveal their feelings, thoughts, and reactions as they face life-threatening situations. First story is about an apparently healthy 35 year-old husband, father, and successful architect who enters hospital for suspected brain tumor. Confirmed diagnosis is followed by surgery, cardiac arrest, and death (see Program 6, Entry C-34D, for nurse's viewpoint). Second story involves an active widow who, after hospitalization, becomes suspicious about the gravity of her situation and is blocked from attempts to talk about her concern by evasive responses and false reassurance from her physician, daughter, son, and friends. Recognizing their discomfort, she discontinues her efforts and, solely with the support of her own faith, faces impending death alone.

34F. Program 6. *Viewpoint: The Nurse.* 89 frames, 26 minutes.
Two personal accounts of nurses involved with dying patients. Story One portrays the range of feelings and reactions experienced by the nurse who provided nursing care for the architect in Program 5 (Entry C-34E); depicts her feelings of helplessness, the overwhelming emotions that were evoked when patient expressed fears of dying, and the frustration and failure she felt upon his death. In the second story, the death of a patient in an intensive care unit provokes intense feelings of sadness and helplessness in the head nurse as she vividly recalls her father's dying and death and her regrets for what she did not do for him. Work conflict is created by nurse's desire to show compassion, project a professional image, and maintain control.

35. *Planting Things I Won't See Flower.* Film, videocassette, color, 26 minutes, rental only, United Methodist Communications, 1976. Distributed by United Methodist Film Service, 1525 McGavock Street, Nashville, TN 37203. (615) 327-0911.

Interview with a dying woman and her family several months before her death from Hodgkin's disease. Conversations with the patient, her husband, and her nine-year-old daughter provide an intimate portrait of a family struggling to meet the demands imposed by a terminal illness, to cope with their own needs and fears, and to find answers to difficult questions.

36. *A Psychosocial Aspect of Terminal Care: Anticipatory Grief.* Audiocassette, 32 minutes, 1972. See Entry C-13 for media details.

Address given by Robert Fulton at a Columbia University symposium in 1971. Content almost identical to Fulton's publication co-authored with Julie Fulton and annotated in Entry A-112.

37. *Psychosocial Aspects of Death.* Film, b/w, 39 minutes, rental only. Produced and distributed by Audio-Visual Center, Indiana University, Bloomington, IN 47401. (812) 337-2105.

Portrays nursing student's involvement with patient readmitted to hospital for leukemia. Depicts the student's struggles with her feelings in her efforts to acknowledge that the patient is dying. Shows the turmoil and distress she experiences when the patient dies unexpectedly and she must cope with facing his death.

38. *Religious Faith and Death: Implications in Work with the Dying Patient and His Family.* Audiocassette, 32 minutes, 1972. See Entry C-13 for media details.

Symposium address by Reverend Carl Nighswonger in 1971. Says his experience with 450 hospitalized dying patients and their families indicates that appropriateness is the key factor in determining whether the dying experience is essentially positive or negative. Presents guidelines for appropriateness, notes how health professionals can be catalysts and facilitators in helping a patient die as a person with dignity. Emphasizes need for health professionals to shift their focus of concern from cure and healing to coping with dying, and discusses how religion/clergy can help the patient find meaning in his dying.

39. *The Right to Die.* A title cited in some film listings instead of the complete title, *ABC News Close-Up: The Right to Die.* See Entry C-1 for annotation.

40. St. Christopher's Hospice: A Living Experience. Audiocassette, 38 minutes, 1975. See Entry C-13 for media details.

A descriptive word tour of this 54-bed London facility for the dying includes conversations with patients, family members, and hospice staff as they tell interviewer Connie Goldman about the loving care and comfort the hospice provides. Descriptions of personal experiences and sharing of feelings evoke word pictures of a loving community where each person is important and each patient is helped to live until he dies.

41. *Soon There Will Be no More of Me.* Film, color, 10 minutes, 1972, rental/sale, Lawrence Schiller. Distributed by Churchill Films, 662 North Robertson Boulevard, Los Angeles, CA 90069.

Dying young mother makes a filmed diary for her daughter, now an infant. Shares inner thoughts and feelings as she tells her story and attempts to communicate her love and values.

42. *A Special Kind of Care.* Film, color, 13½ minutes, 1968, rental/sale, Harvest Films, Inc. See Entry C-5 for distributor.

Gives information about services Cancer Care of the National Cancer Society provides. Dramatizes life situation involving middle-income family with young mother dying of cancer. Depicts impact of illness on family and communication problems that patient, husband, teen-age daughter, and ten-year-old son have as children wonder why their mother, cared for at home, is getting no better. Raises question whether patient and/or children should be told the truth about prognosis.

43. *The Spirit Possession of Alejandro Mamani.* Film, color, 27 minutes, rental/sale, American Universities Field Staff. Distributed by Filmakers Library, Inc., 290 West End Avenue, New York, N. Y. 10023. (212) 877-4486.

Describes an elderly Aymara Indian's struggle against the ills of aging and bereavement -- his grief, loneliness, fears of rejection. Includes English subtitles. A discussion guide accompanies the print.

44. *Stages of Dying.* Audiocassette, 32 minutes, 1972. See Entry C-13 for media details.

Kubler-Ross, in an address given in 1971, tells how her work with dying patients began, and how her first experience with a dying patient, followed by a student seminar, influenced her future work. Indicates what health care givers can learn from patients. Discusses five stages of dying. Explains and gives examples of language patients use–plain English, symbolical nonverbal, and symbolical verbal. Discusses how hope of dying persons differs from that of the healthy, and how dying patients' hope can be supported. Considers denial and how used by health care workers.

45. *Sudden Infant Death Syndrome–After Our Baby Died.* Film, color, 21 minutes, 1975, free loan. Obtain from U. S. Department of Health, Education, and Welfare, Bureau of Community Health Services, Program Services Branch, Parklawn Building, Room 12A-33, 5600 Fishers Lane, Rockville, MD 20852, or from National SIDS Foundation, Room 1904, 310 South Michigan Avenue, Chicago, IL 60604.

Designed "to increase awareness of the trauma and suffering experienced by parents of SIDS babies and to underline the importance of effective parent counseling by the health professionals." Looks at infant's death through the eyes of the bereaved family. Also listed as *After Our Baby Died.*

46. *Talking to Children About Death.* Audiocassette, 57 minutes, 1972. See Entry C-13 for media details.

Informal interview with physician/teacher George G. Williams. Discusses the need for children to participate in situations involving dying and death of persons significant to them. Uses personal life situations to illustrate hazards of attempting to protect children from the realities of dying and death. Suggests children often respond to adult or parental attitudes toward a fact rather than to the fact itself. Believes health professionals must take greater responsibility in helping people adjust their attitudes toward accepting the inevitability of death.

47. *Though I Walk Through the Valley.* Film, color, 30 minutes, 1972, rental/sale. Distributed by Pyramid Films, Box 1048, Santa Monica, CA 90406.

Filmed during the last few weeks of the life of a middle-aged professor dying of cancer. Professor and family discuss their feelings about his illness, impending death, and God.

48. *To Die Today.* Film, b/w, 50 minutes, 1972, rental/sale, Canadian Broadcasting Company, Toronto. Distributed by Filmakers Library, Inc., 290 West End Avenue, New York City, NY 10023.

Presents variety of scenes in keeping with Kubler-Ross's commentary on consequences of institutionalization, attitudes of health care professionals whose focus is on cure and on preserving and prolonging life. Discusses the stages of denial, anger, bargaining, depression, preparatory grief, and acceptance. Interviews 30-year-old man with Hodgkin's disease to illustrate unusual individual who has accepted his condition. In seminar with students that follows interview, students see denial and anger in patient. Kubler-Ross suggests these emotions may be their own.

49. *Until I Die.* Film, videovassette, videotape, color, 30 minutes, rental/sale. Audiocassette, 30 minutes, sale only; WITW-TV. See Entry C-5 for distributor.

Kubler-Ross makes general comments about our death-denying society and the factors that contribute to making dying mechanized and dehumanized. Points out that health professionals who are educated to focus on cure and recovery are not adequately prepared to meet the needs of dying patients. Discusses stages of denial, anger, bargaining, depression, preparatory grief, and acceptance; indicates how health care professionals can go through same stages. Considers special problems in caring for dying children, and discusses importance of hope and ways to support it. Interviews 60-year-old man with cancer before audience. Staff members share their reactions in conference following viewing.

50. *What Man Shall Live and not See Death?* Two-reel film, color, 57 minutes, 1971, rental/sale, NBC Educational Enterprises. Distributed by Films Incorporated, 1144 Wilmette Avenue, Wilmette, IL 60091.

Explores customs and practices surrounding dying and death in the following ways: Kubler-Ross interviews a dying woman; man strolls through cemetery and comments on attitudes toward death and the dead; film-maker tells of decision to use cryogenics for her dead father's body and shows cryogenic process. Scenes from St. Christopher's Hospice in London include an interview with a dying patient and another with Cicely Saunders. In second reel, comments about medical education and its focus on life preservation are followed by glimpses of seminars held for hospital physicians to help them deal with their own feelings about dying and death; two physicians discuss starting and stopping heroic measures. Three clergymen give their respective religious viewpoints; a psychologist is seen working with bereaved children; a widower and his children share feelings about and reactions to the dying and death of a wife and mother; a 77-year-old poet gives his view of life and death; a healthy old woman gives reason for signing a living will; and residents in a home for the aged share their feelings about dying and death. Camera periodically returns to classroom where Robert Neale is lecturing about death.

51. *Whose Life Is It, Anyway?* Film, color, 53 minutes, 1975, rental/sale, Granada Television, Great Britain. Distributed by Euthanasia Educational Council, 250 West 57 Street, New York City, NY 10019. (212) 246-6962.

Intelligent, mentally alert, 35-year-old sculptor Ken Harrison is in a hospital intensive care unit as result of an automobile accident that has left him completely and permanently paralyzed from the neck down. Outraged by his condition, he demands the right to choose between dying with dignity and living, as he is totally dependent on technological life supports and care by hospital staff. His fight for the right to refuse treatment and to be allowed to die, and the care providers' efforts to prevent such action, are dramatically portrayed.

52. *You Are not Alone.* Film, color, 25 minutes, n.d., free loan. Available from United States Department of Health, Education, and Welfare, Bureau of Community Health Services, Program Services Branch, Parklawn Building, Room 7A-20, 5600 Fishers Lane, Rockville, MD 20852, or from National SIDS Foundation, Room 1904, 310 South Michigan Avenue, Chicago, IL 60604.

Looks at sudden infant death through the eyes of families and relatives whose infants were victims of this unexplained and unpreventable syndrome; follows their progression from confusion and anger to understanding and acceptance.

53. *You See I've Had a Life.* Film, b/w, 30 minutes, 1972, rental, Eccentric Circle Cinema. Distributed by University of California, Extension Media Center, 2223 Fulton Street, Berkeley, CA 94720.

Documentary about 13-year-old Paul Hendricks who has leukemia. Shows bright teenager, who likes sports and school, living an average life between hospitalizations. Depicts how family faces crisis with loving concern, tries to share the dying experience, and makes it possible for Paul to die surrounded by his loved ones without medical paraphernalia to keep them apart.

author index

Not listed in this index are authors of reprints that, although listed under citations in Section B, are not annotated in Section A.

subject index